AF824109

How We Age IS A Choice

JOHN P LENHART, MD

Copyright © 2025 by John P. Lenhart, MD

ISBN #: Paperback 978-1-930822-34-4

E-book 978-1-930822-36-8

Audiobook 978-1-930822-37-5

All rights reserved. No part of this book may be reproduced or transmitted in any form or by any means, electronic or mechanical, including photocopying, recording, or by any information storage and retrieval system, without permission in writing from the copyright owner.

This book was printed in the United States of America.

5001-LENH

CONTENTS

5001-LENH

Chapter 8

Chapter 9

Chapter 10

Chapter 11

5001-LENH

DISCLAIMER

This book is not intended to act as a substitute for advice from your personal physician. The information presented in this book is for educational purposes only and not intended to diagnose or treat disease, nor to render medical advice. Before starting any longevity program, please consult your personal physician to determine the appropriateness of that program based upon your personal medical history.

The information in this book was derived from personal experiences of the author, original research, other books on similar subjects, basic research papers, research of other individuals, and anti-aging seminars and lectures at the American College for Advancement in Medicine.

Forward

My previous book, "**Happy life Healthy Aging**", was filled with scientific details. The purpose of this book is to provide you with the basics that are easily comprehended. The supposition being, that if it's simple it would be more accessible in understanding the principles which allow our bodies to work effectively for as long as possible.

We have choices. Aging does not have to be debilitating. Aging can be a pleasant experience so long as we make the choice to keep our body running.

This book is designed to show you how the body compares with ordinary things in our lives, such as cars, houses, or possessions that need to be maintained to get a longer and more serviceable life out of them. Consequently, preventive maintenance matters in all the machines that we possess, including the most important one, our body.

The body is constantly being rebuilt. Our cells die off and new cells are formed. Our brains, muscles, bones, skin, and internal organs all get replaced as new cells are formed. We can influence the health of those systems by what we choose to do physically and mentally. Strong building blocks produce strong houses. Moreover, how the body is maintained makes all the difference in the world in regard to how much serviceable life you will get.

Reality

If we look at the aging global population, and especially of people over 65 years old, by 2050 we will see a huge increase in the number of older people. This population explosion will be staggering.

The Asian population of seniors in 1980 was about 109 million. By 2050 that population is expected to be 948 million. That is an 870% increase in the Asian population of people 65 and older.

Africa and the Middle East had a senior population of about 21 million in 1980. By 2050 the population of seniors is expected to be 198 million people. That will be a 940% increase in this sector of seniors.

South America and the Caribbean population of seniors was about 15 million in 1980. By 2050 the population of seniors over 65 years of age is expected to be 142 million. That also will be a whopping increase of 947%.

Oceana (e.g. the Pacific Islanders and other nearby oceans) had a senior population of about 2 million people in 1980. By 2050 that population in those regions is expected to increase to 11 million, a 550% increase. Also, consider, as space on those islands is limited, they have to import much of their food.

In North America and Europe, the 65 and older senior population was about 113 million in 1980. By 2050, that population is expected to jump to 303 million seniors, a 268% increase.

As you can see by these staggering numbers, the world's senior population may expand beyond sustainability. Who is going to pay for the services when those people cannot take care of themselves? How will this population increase affect all the other people in the future? Currently, my daughter who has traveled to Africa, and knows the situation there, is helping to support one young girl in order for this girl to have the ability to buy food. That is only one person.

If you live in an area of the world where the senior population will eventually explode by 900% then you will have to be totally reliant on yourself. You will most assuredly need to keep your body in good shape, just so that you can survive. If you live in one of the wealthier areas of the world, you will have to do the same thing because your retirement and health benefits may be cut. The question that comes to mind is, will there be enough money to go around to take care of all the sick people that are incapacitated?

How we age is a choice, but healthy aging may also become a necessity for survival. The trick will be to increase our health span instead of just our life span. After all, what good is living longer on a ventilator in a hospital, or being kept alive an extra 12 months taking debilitating chemotherapeutic drugs?

The intent of this book is to help you achieve that very long health span where you can have fun in your old age and with few health limitations.

Introduction

A few years ago, a book called "Passages" was written. It described the stages of life we go through as we pass through this beautiful earth of ours. Our time here is only a fraction of a blink in the grand scheme of things. If you look at the sky, you will see our Milky Way galaxy. This Milky Way Galaxy has about two hundred billion stars just like our sun. Each star has an average of two planets circling it. There are currently estimated to be over 2 trillion observable galaxies like our Milky Way.

Just like an ant cannot comprehend a car, we cannot comprehend such high numbers. Our existence and knowledge of the universe is miniscule.

Our existence is also finite. How we can maximize our potential to get the full benefit of this earth is what this book deals with. I want you to have a happy life and healthy aging. No one can guarantee anything in this life, but by using existing knowledge and observing millions of years of nature, we can try to increase our chances of achieving that healthy aging goal. This is not a trial run; you must think things through and plan what you want to do, then implement that plan in the final trimester of your life.

"How We Age Is a Choice" is my effort, through all the knowledge I have accumulated during my various degrees and clinical experience, to put a cohesive plan together for you that hopefully will maximize your chances of obtaining that goal. Few things in this life happen by chance. You had to put in a lot of effort to get to that stage in life where you are now. In retirement the same rules apply. Having lived in Florida for a long time, I have seen many passages. The health and lifestyle choices people made on those paths made a huge difference in their ability to enjoy the fruits of their labor.

My mission in life now, as a semi-retired doctor, is to outline the principles laid down in this book that will help you succeed in gaining a **Happy Life and Healthy Aging.** There are choices on how you age, so choose wisely.

May you be happy, healthy, wise, prosperous, successful and in love with your life on this earth. Best wishes on your journey.

Dr. John P. Lenhart

CHAPTER 1

Choices

How much do you care about yourself? You have choices. If you care a lot, then you will think hard about what this book says and try to implement some of the concepts presented. If you do not care about your self-preservation, then just go with the flow and let fate handle your retirement years. You have choices.

Recently, on a tour in China, the tour guide explained how young women evaluate men. The guide stated that women make dating choices based on the 5 C's. These criteria must be met by a guy before she even starts considering him as a dating partner or potential mate.

The 5 C' the man needs to possess are: (1) Car, (2) Cash, (3) Condo, (4) College, (5) Career.

These women know that if the above criteria are met, they have a better chance of having a good life with their potential partner.

In retirement communities, most women presumably make similar evaluations. Is the man healthy, is he still able to drive, is he financially sound, can I enjoy life with him, will he be a good companion, so I don't have to live alone, or does he simply want a nurse and a purse?

When we consider car purchases, we do similar evaluations. We look at write-ups about the reliability of the car, maintenance needed, gas mileage, frequency of breakdowns and durability. How long will this car last? Will I have to nurse it and spend a lot of money just to keep it running?

In our lives, we make many choices to meet objectives that we are trying to achieve. If you want to be an engineer, you choose the university that you think has a good engineering program based on reviews. You need to choose the type of engineer you want to become. Will it be a mechanical, civil, or chemical engineer? Or will it be a mining, electrical, computer, or aerospace engineer? Among all those engineering fields, you can choose to subspecialize. In civil engineering, you can become an expert in water resources, or structural engineering, and so on.

On a recent world cruise, I heard an amazing performance of an accomplished accordion player. This young talented musician started playing at age 5 and practiced thousands of hours to develop muscle memory. She had to make choices on whether she would go outside and play with her friends or practice her accordion. When she was in her early twenties, she had to figure out how she could earn a living playing the accordion. She was Chinese and couldn't speak English, so she made a choice to lock herself up for a year and taught herself how to speak English. After one year, being totally immersed in English, she was able to go out and perform to English speaking audiences and started to perform on cruise ships as a one-person band. At times, she was able to make that accordion sound like a full orchestra playing classical music, or, at other times, as a country band playing 'Cotton Eye Joe.' She made a series of choices in her early life that culminated in her becoming a world class performer playing an instrument that few people played. She also learned how to tell jokes in English to connect with the audience. This was such an unusual case, by a determined lady, for a successful career that I had to include it in this book

I could go on detailing all the career choices that we have to make, such as being a teacher, a doctor, a lawyer, mechanic, realtor, software engineer, real estate developer, or beautician. The choices we make early on in life have significant consequences later when we are nearing retirement.

If we make the right choices for ourselves, we will be happy in our lives and fulfilled with what we do, where and how we live, and the lifestyle we have. Everything depends on the series of choices we make throughout life.

How about aging well? You need to make choices early on to keep your body well lubricated and healthy so that it doesn't fall apart on you as you age. These aging choices you make will have a great effect on your ability to enjoy retirement life. You don't want your body to need a nurse and a purse.

It all boils down to instant gratification vs long term benefit. Having a long-term perspective on aging allows for the healthy life you choose. What do you want to be able to do as you age? Do you want to be able to walk longer distances, travel, ride a bicycle, play golf, tennis, pickle ball, get in and out of an RV, take long vacations, and play with the grandchildren? All require physical stamina, and this just doesn't happen by itself. Recently, I saw a discussion on TV about a pill that you take that does all the exercise for you. You don't have to go to the gym or take walks because the pill will cause you to lose weight and gain muscle mass. Sounds Utopian doesn't it, all rewards without any work. Is that how nature works?

There is no such thing as a free lunch, just as there is no such thing as healthy aging without putting some work into it.

It is imperative to have a plan and to work on that plan. At the passenger talent show on my world cruise, a comedian joked, "When I was younger, I had a round butt and a flat stomach. Now that I am older, I have a round stomach and a flat butt." We all know that as we age things seem to drop due to gravity. Your muscles turn flabby, your skin becomes saggy, and your belly drops from your chest to your pelvis and so on. Since this is the normal state of affairs, we have to do whatever we can to mitigate that situation and keep things propped up. We must maintain tone and strength so that we can continue to do the things we want to do.

This is where instant vs delayed gratification comes in. You have choices every day. Do you really need dessert after every meal? Should I order that burger loaded with bacon and cheese, or should I get a salad with extra virgin oil and vinegar or an herb dressing? Do I really need to eat three full meals a day? Or, can I get along with two meals or two meals and a light snack? What does the scale say, what does the body mass indicator, or fat measurement, scale say? What percentage of your body is lean muscle mass vs fat? How far can you walk without running out of breath? What is your VO_2 maximum (the ability to process oxygen that you inhale)?

All those are objective biological measurements of aging. They tell you how old you are physiologically vs chronologically. Your chronological age is measured by the number of years you are old. Your physiological age is the number of things you can still do. Your physiological age may be older than your biological age or younger. It could be equal to a person much older than you, or equal to a person 10 to 20 years younger because you can still do the things that much younger people can do.

If you are a "buy now, pay later" person, you may be reading the wrong book. But if you are the type to save for a rainy day, you have a better chance of reaching your retirement happiness goals. It all boils down to the details, the small choices you make in everyday life.

Liberace, the famous pianist showman, once stated that "If you don't have your health, you cannot enjoy life." Think about it, he was right.

On a recent world cruise, most of the people were in their 70s and 80s. The people that took care of themselves were able to go on the more vigorous tours. They could climb the uneven stairs of the Great Wall of China, they did not need mobility scooters, walkers or canes, they went to the gym regularly, ate more fruits, vegetables and fish, and they looked healthy. The people that did not take care of themselves were, generally, significantly overweight, had to take elevators everywhere, struggled to walk short distances and ate gobs of calorie rich food. You did not see them in the gym. You did, however, see them with heaps of food on their plates at breakfast, lunch, dinners, and even at the late-night buffet.

Both groups of retirees made choices in their life that got them where they were. Both sets of people made the right career and financial choices to be able to go on a world cruise, but they did not make the same health choices for maintaining their bodies. The unhealthy individuals could not enjoy the cruise as well as the healthy passengers because they had physical and health restrictions that most likely were a result of past bad health choices. One of the passengers I knew had a stroke during an excursion, while others had falls, and several others died.

How are healthy or unhealthy choices made? They are made daily in what you choose to do or not do.

Look at your retirement as a Job. Your mission is to stay healthy.

On this world cruise there were many activities to choose from. You could sleep in and have breakfast in bed, or you could get up and do morning stretch, followed by an abs and total body conditioning class. There were also passenger-inspired Zumba-style aerobic sessions, which I liked going to. The aerobics classes were in the same room where the morning chats took place. The morning chat was a question-and answer session from various staff on the ship or guest entertainers. The aerobics classes ran from 8 to 8:30 and the morning chat started at 9 AM.

To get a good seat for the morning chat, passengers would start arriving at 8:20 and watch us do aerobics, looking at us as entertainment. Many of those passengers would have a cup of coffee and sweet rolls. They could have gotten up earlier and participated, but that would have required effort. It's a lot easier to just have a cup of coffee and watch someone else do it than to do it yourself. This one little event is a good example of how daily choices affect our aging. You have a choice to do something beneficial for your body, or a choice to do nothing, or even something harmful to your body and waistline. Excess fat, which is produced from sugar and carbs, must go somewhere. You may even develop insulin resistance and diabetes from all those sweet rolls.

The people on the floor doing aerobics had thinner bellies, better coordination, and greater stamina than the people sitting having a cup of coffee and a sweet role. The coffee sippers could have gotten up and joined us in aerobics, even for 10 minutes, but day after day they just sat there waiting for the morning chat to start.

During my daily piano practice sessions at 6 AM, I would see people walking on the promenade deck. The multipurpose room was located on that deck. This room had a piano in it for church services, and in order to get my practice in, I would have to practice before the room was used for other purposes. Sometimes I would start practicing at 5 AM. To my surprise, between 5 and 6 AM people were starting to exercise by walking the decks at a fast pace. I used to keep the curtain cracked open so that I knew when the sun rose, and that's how I saw the walkers. These were fit people walking briskly and getting their exercise in before the day started. The ship had so many lectures and activities, so the best time for them to exercise was early morning.

One morning, at my Total Body Conditioning class in the gym, a lady came in and watched a small group of us exercise with the instructor, and then left. Later in the day I saw that lady by the elevator and she said, "I watched you in the gym at the exercise class this morning. It looks like fun, do they have that every day?" I replied, "Yes, why don't you come and join us?" She said, "I would, but I have" this and that at that time. This lady had a choice, do something else, alternate doing something else with something healthy, or do something healthy to maintain her body by joining the exercise class. I was surprised that after three and a half months of it being listed in the daily schedule, the lady did not know that that exercise class existed. Coincidentally, she never did come back to join the exercise group.

Inertia is a lot easier than taking action. Unfortunately, our bodies were not designed for inertia and will break down, ache, and squeak much faster if not used, just like our house doors. Our bodies were developed over millions of years to move. In prehistoric societies, Homo sapiens had to walk, run, hunt, and seek shelter to survive. Those that were best at it survived and became modern human beings. This is true of every mammal on earth. Mammals such as lions, horses, cats, dogs, or cows must all seek food while also learning to live without food until they find some. If they didn't have physical and mental stamina, they just perished. The reality is that we need to do the same thing, stay physically strong as we age to survive and thrive.

So, what are the aging choices that allow you to have an enjoyable retirement? There are no guarantees in life, all we can go by are statistics. Based on data collected through numerous experiments, we know that if you do certain things your chances are much better in having that healthy fun-filled life you deserve. You will be able to play pickle ball, go on RV trips, go hiking, and go on more active excursions while on cruises exploring the world. It all boils down to small choices that you make as you go along. They will either force you to be a slave to a continuous schedule of doctor visits and pills, or a master of your life. If you make the right choices, you will have fewer doctors' visits and more fun visits to your favorite activities and destinations.

It all starts in the mind; you must make up your mind to preserve your body. That is not a small task. It is one of the most important tasks that you will undertake as you advance in age. You only have one life and limited time, so use it well.

Any project that you undertake first starts with a plan. That is why in this book I start with the mind. It just doesn't happen by itself, you need to conceptualize what you want, you need to set goals of what you want to achieve, and what state you want to be in five years from now. If you have precise, detailed, written goals as to where you want to be mentally and physically in five years, then you will have a target to shoot for. That target will affect the small decisions you make in your daily life to help you achieve that five-year goal.

In life, change is always constant, nothing stays the same. Your daily choices will need to adapt to change. The results of your choices will, eventually, be measured by how your body looks, how strong you are, how active, how mentally sharp, and ultimately by how you feel.

The more specific and detailed your healthy aging goals are, the greater your chances of obtaining them will be. Write them down and review them each year in January.

On a recent visit to Da Nang Vietnam, one of the passengers went to a stone mason shop where they make fancy gravestones. He told me that he was thinking of having one made here because of excellent craftsmanship and cheaper prices. He is a very nice gentleman that is making choices on how his gravestone will look. After our conversation, I thought about what he did. Looking at and picking gravestones is something I never thought of doing. I guess I'm more focused on prolonging life than worrying about how my gravesite will look. Thinking back on it, I can't recall ever having seen that passenger in the gym?

The focus here needs to be on how we process choices. The choices must be reasonable and achievable. We need to fully understand the consequences of our actions. If someone told you when you were young, "Don't play with firecrackers, you may lose your fingers," would you listen to them? Or would you keep on playing with them because they made a big bang and gave you pleasure? How about if someone told you, "Don't smoke, you may get emphysema where you can't breathe, or even lung cancer." Would you listen to them? Or keep on smoking because you like the way that cigarettes taste, or the way they make you feel, or you can't break the habit?

We know through thousands of research articles that certain foods are not good for us. We can see how societies that change their eating habits because of western fast foods, become less healthy, obese, and start getting the same diseases and cancers of western societies. The data is very clear, yet people choose to ignore it. Just like the firecracker and smoking examples above, people make choices that either keep them out of trouble or slowly start them on trajectories that disable them later in life. We all know of people with diabetes, cardiovascular disease, emphysema, and cancer. How many people do we know are leading healthy active retired lives?

After being on a world cruise, I would guess that at most, twenty percent of the passengers were walking the decks, or going to exercise classes or the gym. Most were sedentary, overweight, and participated in activities most children do in grade school, such as arts and crafts, water coloring etc. They go to lectures that are interesting but not mentally challenging. At breakfast, lunch, and dinner many plates were completely full. They were making small choices daily that either enhanced or diminished their longevity prospects.

On a sea day, one midafternoon, while writing this chapter in the ship's library, a lady in her mid-70s sat down to read a book. I knew this lady well; she grew up on a farm in Wisconsin with many siblings doing regular farm chores. At lunch one day, she proudly told me that she walked all the decks and all the stairs every day. She started out on the bottom floor and did the full length of the ship on both sides and then took the stairs to the next floor until she hit the tenth deck.

The next day she would start on the top floor and go down. When she finishes, she has breakfast. I had run into her many times walking at a reasonably fast pace on my floor and wondered where she was going. Sometimes she would drag her husband along. This lady was thin and full of energy. She was making a daily choice to get out of bed at 6 AM and do her exercise routine. She knew that walking improved her life, and she had the willpower and determination to do it every day that we were at sea. Her husband was one of the early deck walkers I spoke of earlier.

When she got up from her seat at the library, I asked her, "How are you are doing?" She replied, "Everything is great, I had a nice walk, had lunch with Jack, and am looking forward to the show tonight."

People like her are not that common. I saw significantly overweight individuals sitting at the breakfast table eating and chatting for hours. Some ate lunch and dinner at normal times and came back at 10 PM for a night snack at the lido café. Some used a cane and may have had bandages around their ankles because of diabetic microvascular disease and neuropathy.

Both types of people mentioned above make choices daily; those choices will have significant outcomes as they age further. The deck walker will keep on cruising around the world enjoying the various cultural and historical sites, comparing civilizations and wondering how people are so different and yet so much alike. People like her will travel in their RVs exploring the country, visiting national parks, campgrounds, and landmarks. They will go dancing, skiing and play pickle ball. Others will not be able to climb on to the first step of a motor home. They will be tethered to an oxygen tank, or delegated to a nursing home bed, and possibly get bed sores.

The writing is on the wall, you can also see it written on the bellies of people. Those having pendulous bellies with internal visceral fat are in the most danger. This sets you up for a heart attack or stroke. Those external rolls of fat, while they are less dangerous than internal fat, are not good for your looks.

How we age is truly a choice, in more ways than you realize. The choices we make now to maintain our body and mind will have significant effects on how well we age and our ability to enjoy life later.

The following chapters will explain in simple terms the choices that give you the greatest chance of a healthy and contented retirement. I left out all the scientific details that were in my previous book "Happy Life Healthy Aging". I noticed that readers were getting bogged down with science and would put the book down. This book now focuses on the fundamentals and is in simple to understand terms with all the information you need to make wise decisions.

5001-LENH

CHAPTER 2

Choices in Healthy Aging

You're starting to feel a little older, aren't you? You're thinking more often about aging now, especially when you look in the mirror. You compare yourself to friends of your age and secretly see how they measure up to you.

Why do you suppose you feel that way? Is there something inside you that is saying, "There must be something I can do about it?" Is that what made you want to read this book?

Or did a friend tell you that following its suggestions made profound changes in his life.

For whatever reason, the best thing you could have done to help retard the aging process was to pick up and start reading this book. Obviously, you're not the average person who lets fate and the environment rule you and allows your life to slowly degenerate and wither away. Not you. You want to stay active, mentally alert, strong and vigorous. You would like to remain interested in exploring the world and all its possibilities well into your old age and without physical restrictions. You want to *LIVE* and not let the world pass by you, biding your time, until you finally hit the grave.

One good thing about healthy aging is that it is never too late to start. You can begin a longevity program in your 30's, 40's, 50's, 70's, 80's, and even 90's. How do I know that?

Back in the late 70's, I started practicing preventative medicine. Early on, after I had my first doctor's degree, as well as training in acupuncture and nutrition, I began observing what changes people made in their lives that affected them in their later years. Through that process of observation, reading, and attending numerous seminars, as well as seeing thousands of patients, I have been able to deduce certain qualities that are essential in preserving a healthy, vigorous life well into old age.

I have spent a considerable amount of time studying many phases of medicine, traditional as well as non-traditional, and I have observed key components that make a significant difference in how patients age. Also, I have always offered alternative/complementary options for patients' conditions that reduced, and many times eliminated, the need for drugs and invasive surgery. Over the years, I've observed that **many conditions are totally preventable, especially chronic degenerative diseases that plague society today.**

I've also noticed that starting at almost any age, it is possible to reverse the downhill spiral of aging and live a vigorous, healthy lifestyle well into the 80's and 90's. Theoretically, it is possible to maintain an active, healthy lifestyle past 100 or even 120. But, if I said you could be healthy at age 120 or 150, you wouldn't believe me, would you? So, let's not get far-fetched. Let's make things easily understandable and attainable. We want to have a healthy and vigorous lifestyle well into our 80's and 90's, like so many of those world cruise passengers.

I'm certain that there will be things in this book you will believe and others that you will doubt, which is normal in human nature. Things you doubt, you need to research on the internet yourself. The references will be posted on my web site happylifehealthyaging.com. However, do be cautious; information posted on the internet is not necessarily true. Go to the NIH (National Institute of Health) or NCCIH (The National Center for Complementary and Integrative Health) web sites. Other research recognized and peer reviewed journals such as JAMA, Scientific American, Nutrition, Annals of Internal Medicine, Lancet, NEJM and the Cochrane Collaboration are excellent sources. Unless an article has been peer reviewed and gone under intense scrutiny by fellow scientists, it can be very misleading and not accurate. Even peer reviewed articles are sometimes later retracted if the data cannot be replicated by someone else.

So, what are the choices of a happy life and healthy aging? Based upon my clinical experience, following patients throughout their lifetime, completing exhaustive research of the literature, my teaching experience on anti-aging to other physicians, and my extensive training in medicine (both integrative and alternative), as well as in chiropractic, acupuncture, and homeopathy, I have been able to derive key components essential for a beneficial longevity program.

This book has taken key principles and simplified them for easier understanding. If you are interested in more detail about biochemical, hormonal, and specific

5001-LENH

vitamin pathways, you can also read my previous book, "Happy Life Healthy Aging". Also, use Google Scholar for your research. For now, here are the healthy aging choices to assist you.

1. The Healthy Mind Active, Happy and Stress Free. Our psychological input is just as important to our health as our physical input. You choose what goes into your mind, just like you choose how you age. "Garbage in, garbage out," is just as meaningful an expression of our emotions and our psychological wellbeing, as it is in the diet that we eat. Several years ago, Dr. Hans Selye, a prominent Canadian physician, was able to replicate many of the chronic degenerative conditions and diseases that plague us today by stressing animals to the point that their immune systems started breaking down. The result? The animals developed numerous physical ailments. The only variation was the stress placed upon the animals.

We know from experience that our mental well-being plays a large influence on our physical status. Remember, you have choices as to what goes into your mind, and those choices will affect your entire health. I know that whatever I read or watch before I go to sleep affects my dreams and how restful I sleep. If I read scientific research, I will be dreaming about science or seeing patients all night. If I read or watch the news, I will have disturbing dreams throughout the night since no news is good news. To get a good night's sleep, just listen to some music, read a pleasant story, or watch a funny movie. After all, laughter is the best medicine for insomnia.

2. Physical Activity and Exercise -Through my experience as a preventative-minded physician, I've seen numerous patients at death's door, pale, weak, and frail, who then, through physical activity and exercise, totally reverse that status. They become vigorous, active, clear-thinking senior citizens with good muscle tone, agility, and stamina. Numerous studies throughout the world have shown that **physical activity can significantly reduce all disease processes**, including cancer, and at the same time increase our life span, as well as greatly enhance our quality of life and health span. If physical activity was a drug, it would surpass any drug on the market today for its health benefits.

3. Caloric Restriction – Since 1991, the incidence of obesity in the United States has tripled. SUGAR created FAT is winning, making a lot of corporations very wealthy. **The price to our health that high fructose corn syrup plays is catastrophic.** There are scores of diseases associated with obesity and overweight conditions. These diseases, the diseases of western societies, are gradual in onset, rob us of our youthfulness, and gradually induce inactivity, chronic diseases, immobility, mental sluggishness and death. There are numerous well-documented studies that show that **caloric restriction** is one of the healthiest lifestyles for promoting longevity, mobility, and mental acuteness. **As a nation, we're eating ourselves to death.** If this process doesn't stop, we'll be unable to afford to pay for the chronic conditions we will suffer in our lifetime. And we will suffer in misery in our old age.

The good news is that this obesity cycle can be reversed. You can regain good health, at the same time improving your life quality and longevity

4. Clean Out/Detoxify Your Body – Over the years, the body accumulates thousands of toxins that it can only partially eliminate or not eliminate at all. These toxin leave residue that slowly accumulate in the body, clogging up our system and preventing us from metabolizing and working properly. **The gradual toxic biological and chemical sludge that accumulates in our systems slowly bogs down our chemical and electrical processes that cause our body to function normally.** This interference eventually leads to Metabolic Syndrome, the chronic diseases prevalent in today's society, such as diabetes, cardiovascular disease, circulatory problems, stroke, Alzheimer's disease, cancer, arthritis, and numerous other chronic conditions. Toxins are stored in fat cells and the more fat cells you have, the more undesirable chemicals you can store.

5. Happy things to do in Healthy Aging – In order to be happy, we have to do activities that bring us joy. Happy things increase our endorphins, the little pleasure chemicals in our brain. To truly live means to enjoy life to its fullest and fulfill our passions. This chapter discusses possible activities to pursue that we had no time for in our working years and expose you to activities you never thought of. New activities and new experiences all contribute to new brain growth.

6. Vitamins, Minerals, Herbs, and Anti-Oxidants

(This chapter has been significantly modified from my previous book for easier understanding, if you want to learn the scientific details, you may want to read "Happy Life Healthy Aging")

In the 1970's when I was practicing preventive medicine (known as holistic medicine at that time), other doctors scoffed at the money patients were "wasting" on vitamins and minerals. I knew the data was out there. I read basic research from the 1930's and 40's. However, the majority of the medical community was not aware of it and stated that you got all the vitamins and minerals you needed from the food you ate. Taking anything else in addition was a waste of money. Well, how times have changed. Nowadays you see vitamins and minerals constantly advertised on television. Now there's even a going consensus that our food is devoid of necessary vitamins and minerals due to the depletion of our soil and genetic (GMO) modification of the food itself. Did you know that grasshoppers are dying at an alarming rate? Calcium, magnesium and other elements are diminishing in grasslands making the grasses less nutritious so grasshoppers are dying due to malnutrition.

Over forty years after I first recommended vitamins and minerals, the mainstream medical community slowly started to change its opinion on the need for supplementation because the public demanded it, there are well designed studies available now. That public has found that by supplementing daily food intake with necessary vitamins and minerals, they may feel better and they want to prevent some of the ailments of modern society by giving their bodies' optimized nutrition. Antioxidants have been found to prevent free radical damage. Thirty years ago, no one ever heard of free radicals, which destroy our cells slowly. The more we learn about the body, the more we realize that we need proteins and fats, specific vitamins, minerals and essential fatty acids in our foods or through supplementation for optimization of our health.

7. **Hormone Replacements** – Human growth hormone (HGH) and other naturally occurring hormones have only recently been used on an off label basis to enhance the appearance of youth and vitality. The original studies done in the early 1990's by Dr. Dennis Rudman documented the antiaging effects of growth hormone on our muscles, fat tissue, and overall appearance and energy and stamina. Growth hormone decreases with age. Lack of growth hormone in older people is associated with sleep deprivation Sleep deprivation is associated with memory loss and Alzheimer's disease. It's a vicious cycle, but there is hope,

Exercise. Exercise has been shown to increase growth hormone and virility naturally. The only trick is, you have to do it.

Natural hormone replacements for postmenopausal females and some for males trickled into mainstream medicine and the media. However, newer studies advise caution with total body hormone replacements. The risks may outweigh the benefits. Local applications of hormones such as estrogens, has been shown to be effective. It's best to talk to your endocrinologist or gynecologist before starting hormonal augmentation or replacement. (This topic is covered in greater depth in my "Happy Life Healthy Aging" book and in endocrine specific books)

8. Nutrients - The old saying, **"Garbage in, garbage out,"** couldn't hold truer in our biological systems. **What we take in is related to what we get out.** If we consume foods poor in nutrients, the building blocks that build our body are going to be very, very poor. Poor building blocks in our cells, bones, nerve tissues, and muscles make them very fertile for disease processes. This decreased immunity increases our susceptibility to various diseases and even cancers. What held true for the three little pigs and the big bad wolf in the book "The Three Little Pigs", holds true for our bodies. The house the pig built out of brick withstood the huffing and puffing of the big bad wolf. He survived. The houses built of straw and wood the wolf blew over and he ate those pigs. Just think about it: Doesn't cancer eat us up just like the wolf ate the pigs in the weak houses? What kind of house do you want to have? The stronger your immune system, the more resistance you have to chronic diseases.

9. Happy Mind, Healthy Aging -Visualization and laughter therapy have even been used for cancer treatment with success. Reduced stress, happy thoughts, happy relationships, love, and plenty of time for play are essential for healthy human beings and prolongation of life. I have had friends who were big executives in corporations with their own private jets tell me, "I got out of this rat race. If I would have stayed in, I would be dead like the rest of my friends."

They are now leading happy retired lives in Florida, playing as much as possible and enjoying life, whereas all their friends are dead. **Happy thoughts and things we do while being socially engaged, are essential for longevity.**

In the following chapters, I will go over the key choices for a happy life and healthy aging. I will give you specific dietary recommendations, exercise regimens, and many other useful hints that may help **prolong your life and increase your quality of life. You will realize that "how we age is a choice".**

Chapter 3

A Healthy Mind:

Active, Happy, and Stress-Free

Warning – this chapter is repetitious, but then all learning is based on repetition.

It's five o'clock in the morning. My mind is working at a feverish pace to come up with a proper title for this chapter. Yes, I had many possibilities written down, but few of them had the spirit of what I am about to tell you. Finding the right word is oftentimes more difficult than you think.

Can you remember how difficult it was for you to tell someone for the first time that you loved them? You were sweating bullets, weren't you? How would that person react? Were you going to be accepted? After all, you were feeling totally vulnerable, weren't you?

But your mind and spirit were ready for a new experience. You were willing to risk it for a greater gain. The promise of total ecstasy and invulnerability, of being on Cloud Nine where nothing else mattered except you and your partner, of high emotions, and the possibility of togetherness. The feeling of love is a very powerful emotion. It can move mountains or part the sea, and even make you feel invincible.

I can still remember many, many, many years ago when I was in seventh or eighth grade, talking to a clergyman. I asked him what made people happy. His response was, **"In order to be happy in life, you have to give more than what you get."** For a twelve-year-old, that concept was rather difficult to comprehend. I thought and thought and thought about it.

How could you survive if you gave more than what you got? It was impossible to do that. You'd end up with a negative balance. You'd be in a hole. After a while, I figured it out, and guess what? He was right. The more you give, the more you get. Whatever good deeds you do come back to you a thousand-fold. What goes around comes around.

You must have heard these statements sometime in your life. Have you ever put any thought behind them? Let me tell you one thing. People who follow these sayings are happy, alert, and stress-free into a very, very, very old age.

There is a power in the universe that keeps track of things. It keeps track of your good thoughts and your bad thoughts, your good intentions and your bad intentions. It is a life force of energy and creativity and your goodness towards humanity.

My mother had that powerful life force. She was kind to others and made people feel good. She was always cheerful. I almost never heard her complain. She was a true friend to all her pals. I have never seen anyone else have as many true friends as she did.

She had both young and old friends. Former bosses were friends. College students were friends. She had friends of different religions. As a matter of fact, after she died, she was baptized into a totally different religion because they valued her so much that they wanted to be assured she went to heaven. Now, those are true friends. People who worry about your soul, even after you're dead, wanting to make sure you made the right choice in religion.

She had a tremendous life force inside her, a spirit that influenced everyone for the better. I have pictures of her camping out in the gorgeous canyons and painted deserts of Utah, going on hiking trips with university students considerably younger than herself. She loved to sing, dance, have fun, get together with people, and volunteer her free time for whatever was needed. She made people feel good.

On lectures at adult living facilities, I would always find people who were like her. They were the ones smiling, attentive, bright, bushy-tailed, and cheery-eyed. They were interested in life. They had keen minds. They could follow my lectures and ask intelligent questions. They smiled a lot. They made my trip to their retirement home worthwhile. Those were people in their late eighties, nineties and even over a hundred. Many of these kinds of people live in the St. Petersburg / Tampa Bay, Florida, area as they love to come to warm climates to retire.

When I asked Activities Directors about them, they tell me these men and women have the best health and the least number of ailments. They frequently inform me that those over a hundred are in much better physical shape than some in their seventies who are always complaining, worrying, and predicting that bad things are going to happen. And believe it or not, bad things do end up happening to them.

Many of the oldest ones have a great attitude toward life. They take things one day at a time and they enjoy things profusely. They always have. They live life fully and it's an adventure for them. They don't worry, just as that song declares, "Don't worry, be happy." They look forward to new things in their life, new activities and maybe future travel plans. Some of the younger retirees talked about their past and didn't look forward to any new adventures. They complained a lot and seemed old, while the older active ones seemed young.

Jessie, a spry 94-year-old that I interviewed in Newfoundland, Canada, told me, "Don't sweat the small stuff." When I met this thin, attractive, well-dressed lady in the adult living facility she lived in, I was truly impressed by all the stacks of large print crossword puzzle books she had next to her rocking chair. She said, "You've got to keep your mind going, because without your mind you have nothing."

She liked living there because of all the friends she had there. Friends were important to her, and she always had lots of friends throughout her life. Her husband was a fisherman, and she would help him out whenever he came home from a trip. She would also gather the firewood, chop it up herself, and do a lot of physical work at home while her husband went out cod fishing. They ate the food they grew or fished in the ocean. For entertainment she would get together with friends to socialize and have tea and cakes.

During our conversation I asked her what she liked to do for fun. She stated that she liked to dance. Suddenly a glimmer came into her eye as she reminisced about an old boyfriend from another town that used to take her dancing. She lost contact with him, as he had moved away, but she still talked about him fondly as if it were yesterday. Those passionate moments of dancing on the dance floor with a boyfriend seventy-five years ago were as clear to her today as they were then.

What I noticed from this very alert 94-year-old lady was that she was actively participating in her longevity program. She used to walk quite a lot until one day she tripped and fell, breaking her hip. She realized that to enjoy life at that age, she had to keep her mind stimulated by doing those crossword puzzles. She said that she didn't eat a lot, just enough to keep her going. Food wasn't a top priority in her life; having friends, being active and staying mentally engaged was more important to her. Jessie had inner happiness, peace of mind, and a warm friendliness about her that everyone loved.

Kindness, inner happiness, peace of mind, and a strong desire to give of yourself are the most important longevity attributes that you can have.

By now you must be saying, "Oh how sweet, but where's the beef?" The "beef" is sandwiched inside your skull. It's all in your mind.

You have free will.

You can decide from this day on that you will have a happy mind. You will turn your greatest adversity into your greatest asset by not letting it get the better of you. You will make lemonade out of lemons. You will make people feel wonderful around you and be happy that they are alive because of your presence. You are going to be a positive person, having as much fun as possible, while doing as much good as possible for the people around you, be it your spouse, your children, your grandchildren, great grandchildren, your neighbors, people in your church, synagogue, or mosque, as well as for the animals and plants around you.

You need to be kind to nature. Every little plant has feelings, and that has been proven repeatedly in numerous biological experiments. Those plants for which you have happy thoughts towards, and chat to, will grow well and thrive, whereas the plants you dislike will shrivel away faster and die, even though they get the same amount of sunlight, water, and nutrition.

Your thoughts influence everything around you. You possess a longevity mind.

Did you know that in January 2000, specifically in that first month, there were numerous deaths in New York? I remember reading about it in the newspaper. The statistics were compared observing the death rate at the beginning of the year 2000. Many, many people had chosen to live for the new millennium. They chose to live! Then, once they got there, they said, "Okay, it's time to let go," and they died.

A friend of mine, a nurse that later became a realtor, died recently. She was a bubbly person. She waited until her relatives were there at her side. About ten minutes after the last one arrived, she died. My mother did the same thing. I flew back from Mexico to be at her side, sitting next to her, holding her hand, and talking to her. Within six hours, she took her last breath and died, peacefully and happy.

Your mind controls your biological functions. Your mind controls your hormone levels. Your mind controls your spirit. Your mind controls your anti-aging processes. "Smile and the whole world smiles with you. Cry and you cry alone." It is all in your mind.

By now, you must be saying, "Dr. Lenhart, this isn't a motivational book. This is a book about healthy aging." Guess what? This is one of the choices you make for healthy aging, your mental attitude. How sharp your mind is, and what you do with your mind, determines how well and how long you are going to live. It also determines your quality of life; how happy you are.

If you're not happy, get out there and start doing volunteer work. Help people who are in need, and you'll find out how lucky you truly are. Go out to nursing homes, hospitals, and children's centers. Become a mentor. Assist in an animal shelter, or even help a poor dog or cat find a new home.

How about a child that is in need, without parents, aimlessly wandering around this world not knowing which direction to head, constantly getting in trouble. Get involved and give a hand. When you help other people you will be helping yourself. Do a variety of things, not just one. A mind needs to be constantly stimulated to stay young.

The older theories about aging used to be that the mind, within its lifetime, generally started losing brain cells and atrophying. If you look at an MRI or CT scan taken when you are older, you will see a lot more fluid-filled spaces and less density in the brain matter. Everyone thought that was a natural progression in aging, until recently when these old theories were re-evaluated. You see, when they initially studied brains, a lot of the brains they studied had brain diseases such as senility and Alzheimer's disease. They did not include in the studies the brains of active, mentally alert adults. They made assumptions that everyone's brains degenerated and atrophied. Those assumptions were wrong. How could Einstein have been active in mathematics well into his old age? How could Linus Pauling have run his research institute in his older years? These people stayed mentally alert and engaged. Recently, at a folk festival, I met a university professor of social anthropology who plans on working till he is eighty.

You want to know a memory enhancement secret? The more education you have, either formal or self-taught, the greater are your chances of staying mentally alert as you age because of your inquisitive nature about life. You will be stressing your neurons and forming new dendrites. You may be saying, "What are you talking about?" Let me back-track.

Your brain has 86 billion cells called neurons or nerve cells, which have stems attached to them. Those stems have very small branches coming off them, and those branches have even smaller branches coming from them called dendrites. Each cell can make thousands of connections. The more densely packed your dendrites are, those tiny little twigs coming off the nerve cells, the greater your ability to make connections. The more education you have, the more you have proliferated those dendrites, and the wider variety of activities you have done and interests you have engaged in, the greater will be the density of your dendritic cluster.

One important thing, you need variety. When you get older, you get crystallization of dendritic patterns. That means that whatever you've been doing all your life, you will still be good at it. For example, a great composer in his nineties will likely be a greater composer because of his wisdom, knowledge, and experience. However, other capabilities diminish. The composer will be good at composing and that's all. Other things are going to be lacking. Variety in activities, variety in living environments, and variety in mental stimulation will keep your dendrites sprouting and keep you mentally alert. In my RV travels, I ran into a solo woman traveler that told me, "At home, everything is always the same. When I'm on the road, I always have new experiences and I need to figure out how to get from place to place, where to shop, where to camp. I must figure out my basic day to day survival, which is automatic at home."

A great musician can play music well into old age. Music is a mental stimulant and is very important in our anti-aging program. I believe it has something to do with the pleasure sensors in our brain. When you are constantly stimulating your pleasure sensors, your mind will be happy and continue to thrive.

In St. Petersburg, Florida, there is a Kids 'n Kubs baseball team where the men are in their eighties playing baseball with vigor, running well, catching and throwing the ball adeptly. They crystallized those activities well throughout their life and can perform them into their old age. Unknowingly, they also improved their mind by physical activity. As well, they increased their blood supply and kept neurons alive.

Let's get into some basic research. Some rat studies were performed to determine how the brain reacted to different stimuli. The first set of rats were locked up in their cages (let's call them condominiums). They would basically walk around inside their four walls (let's call it the living room, kitchen, and bedroom) and didn't do much else.

When these rats died, their brains were dissected and evaluated for dendritic density, trying to find out how many nerve cell connectors they had. It was found, over time, the number of nerve connectors diminished. Their brains got smaller. They were quite content to be in their rat condominium, within their four walls, not doing much of anything. They died with a smaller brain and that was it.

They took another group of rats and changed their environment. Every day they put them in a very exciting environment, a huge box with a lot of different toys that these rats could climb in and out of and explore. They could interact with other rats. "How are you doing this morning? Having fun exploring this environment? Isn't it a beautiful day? Look at this old sock and shoe we can get into."

They had a wonderful time. Then they were put back in their cages. The next day, they were taken out again and put into a box in which all the furniture had been rearranged. Different toys were there for them to play with, so they had a stimulating new environment every time they got out of their condominium.

When it finally came time to see their maker, the rats' brains were sliced up. Guess what the researchers found? These rats had the brains of young rats, full of dendrites. They didn't age at all. They had anti-aging brains.

Mental stimulation allowed them to stay young. They got out, they got involved. They were busy with a variety of things and every day was different, a challenge. They became mentally, aesthetically, physically, and socially stimulated. They met with each other, did things, interacted, and explored. They got out of their four-wall condominiums and became interactive with the rest of the world.

You're saying to yourself, "Well, that makes sense. Mental stimulation and new environments kept them mentally alert. So where do those baseball players fit in?" That's what these researchers thought, although they were not dealing with baseball players, they were dealing with rats. So, they gave another set of little rats a gym in their confined environment. Every day those rats, instead of just sitting around in their cages looking at their four walls, were given a treadmill wheel. These rats got in there and started doing exercises. They ran that wheel in circles and that thing kept them going for hours. They got a good cardiovascular workout.

When it was time for them to be sacrificed, their brains were sliced into little pieces and guess what? They, too, had an increased dendritic pattern, or increased connectors in their brains. Their brains stayed young. The increased physical activity kept their minds young. Even though they didn't have an environment as stimulating as the other rats, they had increased exercise, which was enough to increase the blood flow to the brain. Physical exercise also stimulates the nerve endings, then they don't die due to lack of use.

Atrophy does not occur when you are physically or mentally active. Maybe that explains the perfect shape, both mentally and physically, of my elderly neighbor who walked several miles a day, although it probably didn't hurt that he was also writing poetry and trading stocks.

Pets also seem to make people younger. I remember seeing documentaries on people with amazing dogs and cats. They took their pets to children's hospitals and nursing homes, where everyone perked up. They livened up, became interactive, and they all loved petting these animals. Even people in wheelchairs who were inanimate, just sitting there, suddenly became active and involved with these pets.

Pets, such as cats and dogs, seem to stimulate the brain and influence the pleasure sensors in our brains, which I believe aid in longevity. Sick children do better around these animals. Feeble, older adults respond and become younger again. There is a magic quality to pets that helps keep us young in old age.

If you have a dog, it makes you go out every day for a walk, two or three times a day, which you normally would not do. It makes you care for something, and a dog gives you a tremendous amount of love, affection, and companionship. Cats are totally different creatures' altogether. They give you a tremendous amount of company, love, and physical interaction through their mannerisms, various moods, and playfulness. They are also extremely easy pets to care for. I call them pocket pets.

All you must give them is food, water, and a litter box, which you clean once a week. So, if you are active in doing sports, going to the gym, doing all kinds of activity, you may want to consider a cat because they are a lot less work to care for. I have had both and I'll tell you, that dogs were a lot more work.

You need to be very careful about the kind of pet you choose because dogs and cats are a long-term commitment. If you are very active and go away frequently on trips, or take long cruises, then having a dog that needs to be walked twice a day can become expensive. You either must kennel them or hire a dog sitter. Taking pets to hotels, restaurants, and across international borders can be a problem also. So think hard before you get a pet that can potentially limit your lifestyle. You do not want to become a caregiver to a pet and limit your lifestyle in the years when you can still be highly active, traveling, and enjoying the world. How are you going to take a two week or four-month cruise? A man at the pickle ball court on the cruise ship told me, "I don't get it; people give up traveling just to take care of their pets." Does it make sense to give up the time you have left in this world to take care of an old pet? By the time the pet dies, you may be too old to do anything. At a much older age, when you are less active, pets may become a desirable choice for companionship.

Let us get back to basic research. We are getting a little carried away. By now, you must be following my train of thought and drawing conclusions on my analogies. Fine. But what is the best combination?

In my book, Happy Life Healthy Aging, I spoke of a hormone called cortisol. It is a stress hormone released when the body and mind are under prolonged or tremendous stress. It is a destructive hormone. It ages you rapidly, destroys your brain cells, and causes damage to your tissues. Have you ever seen anyone who has been on Cortisone for any period? They puff up. Sometimes their bones get very frail and brittle, and they break or degenerate. Other organ systems start to fail. Well, that's what stress does to you.

Stress increases the cortisol level, which, over time, destroys our bodies. Mental and emotional stress is a tremendous aging factor. It causes us to age prematurely and die early.

Since increased stress is health-destroying, a reduction of stress must be an important component in your healthy aging program. Like Jessie said, "Don't sweat the small stuff." During a coffee chat on my world cruise, while interviewing a couple, the wife of a top manager stated that what she liked the most about her husband was that he stayed calm when problems occurred. He did not get upset about many things. When he was asked how he stayed so calm, he said, "If it's not a permanent change, get over it and move on."

The more of a stress-free environment you can create around yourself, the happier you'll be and the healthier you'll be.

At this point, it would be a suitable time to discuss the taking of a nap, and the importance of getting a good night's sleep to reduce stress. Lack of sleep increases our cortisol level, the stress hormone, and is associated with insulin resistance and Alzheimer's disease. There are many good books written on the importance of sleep and I would suggest reading some of them.

You must have used the term, "I'll sleep on it," in your life. The reality is that "I'll sleep on it" works. The brain needs rest to filter your daily thoughts, clean out beta amyloid and tau proteins, which are associated with Alzheimer's disease, and to do vital neuronal housecleaning. Sleep is also necessary to heal our emotions. You can be upset one day, and then feel calmer about things the next day after a good night's sleep.

Without sleep, you would die. **Sleep deprivation is a silent killer**, and as we get older we need a lot more sleep. The problem is, for some of us, as we get older it becomes harder for us to sleep. Lack of growth hormone in our system may be the culprit. This is yet another reason why exercise is so important, because exercise increases growth hormones in our bodies.

Naps are an important part of our essential sleep. We need about seven to eight hours of sleep per day for our body and brain to function properly. REM sleep, the rapid eye movement component, is the last part of our deep sleep cycle just before we wake up. As we go to sleep, our brain waves gradually slow down until we reach a deep sleep. After deep sleep, the waves gradually speed up again at the end of the cycle. Those dreams that we try to remember are occurring in the REM phase at the tail end of that cycle. If we are woken up when we are in deep sleep, we feel drugged. We are tired and unable to concentrate. That is why you need to have a full REM sleep cycle if you want to get restful sleep. The entire sleep cycle is about an hour and a half, 90 minutes, but it can vary slightly from person to person.

How do we take a nap? We take a nap in stage one of our sleep cycle. In this stage, which usually lasts about 20 minutes, we have not entered deep sleep yet and can be awakened without feeling groggy. We still get the benefit of mental and physical rest without disturbing our deep sleep cycle. Thomas Edison, the inventor of the light bulb, was able to function quite well taking multiple naps as he worked on his light filament experiments all day and all night.

For me to function fully in the evening, I need that afternoon nap. For a short non-REM sleep, I set my cell phone countdown alarm for 24 minutes and go to sleep. The reason that it's 24 minutes instead of 20 is because I give myself four minutes to fall asleep. Usually, I fall asleep in a couple of minutes. Some people have trouble falling asleep, and their mind will wander, but they do get rest in that time frame.

If you set your timer for 45 or 60 minutes, you may end up waking up in deep sleep, feeling groggy and sleepy for a while. You may not be able to think clearly, because your brain will want to be in a deep sleep and does not want to be woken up. If you want a deeper, more restful sleep, then set your timer for a full REM cycle which is about 90 minutes. If you are awakened during deep sleep, reset your timer for another 90-minute sleep cycle.

To find out how long your sleep cycle is, set a timer for 90 minutes when you want to take a long nap, while at the same time start a timer on a stopwatch or on your phone. Before you close your eyes, say to yourself, "I want to sleep for 90 minutes."

If you naturally wake up before the 90 minutes are up, write it down. If you are groggy, then increase the timer by 5 minutes and see if you feel rested afterward. By monitoring your sleeping times for one cycle, you will be able to determine the length of your normal cycle and set your alarm clock accordingly whenever you want to take a nap. This also helps in determining what time to set your alarm based on when you go to sleep so that you do not end up being woken up in the morning in the middle of a sleep cycle then go out driving in your car. This would be dangerous. By knowing your sleep cycle time, you will know how long to set your timer for a full REM nap and for what time to set the morning alarm based on when you went to sleep.

On the cruise, I took daily naps while out on sea days. I discovered that I usually woke up in less than 90 minutes, and I was fully rested. My alarm was set for 90 minutes but I woke up before that. On land, I seem to require the full 90 minutes.

Now you are saying, "But Dr. Lenhart, you started out this chapter on the subject of love. What's love got to do with it?" The answer is everything. It is about mental attitudes, emotions, and mental stimulation.

Love is the most potent emotion in the universe. The more you can be in a state of love, the happier and healthier your mind is going to be. It could be love for your spouse, love for your pet, for your neighbor, for the work you do, love of a hobby or love of a sport. The more love you can add, the better your life is going to be.

Let's put things into more concrete terms. A while ago, I was lecturing to a group of Optimists. For their appreciation of my lecture on nutrition and chelation therapy, they gave me a plaque called The Optimist Creed, which reads:

The Optimist Creed

Promise Yourself

To be so strong that nothing can disturb your peace of mind.
To talk health, happiness and prosperity to every person you meet.
To make all your friends feel that there is something in them.
To look at the sunny side of everything and make your optimism come true.
To think only of the best, to work only for the best, and to expect only the best.
To be just as enthusiastic about the success of others as you are about your own.
To forget the mistakes of the past and press on to greater achievements of the future.
To wear a cheerful countenance at all times and give every living creature you meet a smile.
To give so much time to the improvement of yourself that you have no time to criticize others.
To be too large for worry, too noble for anger, too strong for fear, and too happy to permit the presence of trouble.

I thought that was a wonderful creed for the Optimist International Organization. It reminds me of a quote from Marjorie Hertz, a ninety-eight-year-old woman living in Naples, Florida. I frequently recite it to other doctors in my lectures on physical activity and anti-aging. Her motto?

"Smile awhile and while you smile, another smiles, and soon there are miles and miles of

smiles, and life's worthwhile because you smiled."

Aren't those quotes wonderful? Just think, if you are always smiling at other people, you are creating good will, and that smile gets carried on and on to other people, passing on good karma to the universe. Remember, what goes around comes around. It's going to come back to you many-fold. It's going to make your life richer. It's going to reduce your aging process. It will add love to your life.

A good mental attitude, for which a smile is very important, is one of the best stress reducers out there.

Remember how I talked about cortisol levels increasing stress and your mind losing its cells and your body deteriorating? You can avoid that by smiling. You can avoid that by not letting anything disturb you. You can avoid that by having peace of mind. By talking health, happiness, and prosperity to every person you meet.

Whenever I have a chance to learn from my patients about aging and longevity, I jump at the chance. Recently, a hair stylist came in as a patient. I found out that she worked in several adult living facilities, which I thought was quite a niche market for a beautician. I asked her about her observations of her older clients, questions primarily about their health, alertness, and what type of clients they made.

When I questioned her about the young/old and the old/old, she stated without hesitation that the young/old, that is, people in their nineties or older, are in better shape many times over than people twenty years younger than themselves because they have a much better attitude. They talk about prosperity and health. They talk about happiness and the joy of life.

About doing things and being involved. They take one day at a time and live it to the fullest.

Meanwhile, those who were always talking about their bad health, how rotten things are, always worried about things and how they were going to fall and break their hips, talking about the misery of others and complaining - believe it or not, their predictions came true. Those people did die younger.

One interesting observation she told me about was that the ninety- and hundred-year-olds she did hair for were far more active, walked better, and had a much better attitude about life than the seventy-five- to eighty-year-olds. She also said their minds and memories were better. They were more resilient, could overcome setbacks better, and were much more pleasant to deal with than the sickly younger population. These older patients seemed to live for the moment, enjoyed life, and overcame obstacles through a positive mental attitude and an active lifestyle.

What your mind can perceive, it will achieve. If you perceive negative thoughts, emotions, and events, then the universe gives it to you. You develop poor health. You may end up having all kinds of problems. Those who smile and talk about health, prosperity, and joy, generally avoid those problems because they have a great weapon in their healthy aging arsenal working for them, their mind and attitude.

I remember seeing a story about an eighty-nine-year-old woman who got a degree from Harvard. It took her sixteen years to get it, but she got it. Even at age eighty-nine, you can still sprout new dendrites by stimulating your mind. You're less likely to forget where you left the keys, or whom you talked to five minutes ago. You can stay mentally alert and sharp just by exercising your mind. It's a potent anti-aging tool. You exercise your mind by using it. If physical exercise increases the oxygenation of the brain, then mental exercise increases the proliferation of the brain cells. **You can improve your mind**.

Many people who have had a great long-term memory end up with a poor short-term memory when they get older. The long-term memory is sort of fixed in your hard drive, which is another part of your brain, and your short-term memory is in your RAM, as in the random memory in your computer. You can increase your RAM by mental stimulation.

Old people oftentimes just love to talk about old events. Those events are impregnated in the hippocampus, a part of the brain that stores that older data which connected to your emotional experiences, and which the brain decided was important to keep. The short-term memory in the cortex is very fluid. It comes and goes. It decreases with age because it's not used. It is not continuously stimulated.

So, what is your job? Your job is to increase the RAM in your computer mind, constantly forcing it to be upgraded. You do that by mental enhancements such as mind games. Remember the Mankato nun study where the nuns donated their brains to science. In the autopsy, it was found they had the brains of young people, even if they were ninety years old, because they were continuously playing mind games such as Jeopardy, theological treatises, crossword puzzles, and so on.

I remember watching a show of an older chess champion who was very competitive, even in his old age, because he was constantly stimulating his mind trying to outwit his opponents. Card games are also good, as are complex jigsaw puzzles, which give you spatial orientation. Also, there are now a host of computer games being developed to enhance memory retention, especially recent memory. Recent memories are important in the activities of daily living.

Experts for a courtroom may be specialists who do one thing only and study one thing only rather than having a varied knowledge base of information. That's great for the courtroom, but that single focus knowledge doesn't do much to keep you young; other areas of your brain will shrivel up.

The more things you study, and the more you do, the younger your mind will be. You have a quest for knowledge. You enjoy variety. You have an anti-aging mind. When you get older, you will be as sharp as a tack. As long as you keep feeding that mind new information, it will continue to grow. At least, your mental acuity will not deteriorate. Learning new things on a variety of subjects will keep your mind constantly stimulated and will increase the RAM in your memory circuits. The cortex of your brain will be forced into action. When that happens, your overall memory will improve. Your short-term retention will improve. You will not be as forgetful and will be able to multitask again.

I have noticed that my chelation patients, when they had chelation therapy with all the vitamins added, their short-term memory improved. They didn't have to write as many notes. Overall, they were mentally more competent. I believe that the result is primarily due to increased circulation to the brain and increased mental stimulation. Exercising alone will increase endorphins, make you feel better, and increase the oxygenation to the brain, giving you greater capacity. This increased capacity needs to be exploited through mental stimulation, through learning new things.

Go back through your life and think of all the things that you have ever been interested in. Make a list. Be creative. Go back to your early childhood. What turned you on? What did you like? Then go decade by decade. Try to recollect the milestones in your life.

People think life is a series of milestones in which they put flags that they can remember things by. I use dates, such as how old I was in a certain year. It's easy for me since I was born in an even-numbered year. I figure out how old I was when something was happening in my life. So, when they mention a certain event in history, I can recall that age and what I was doing in that period. It gives me a benchmark.

Think of your benchmarks. Write them down. What were you interested in? What kind of things did you want to achieve? Were you interested in a particular musical instrument, writing poetry, a particular sport, or a particular activity that you never quite got around to doing? Perhaps you wanted to learn how to quilt, or paint, or write but never had the time. You wanted to become good at horticulture and learn all about different plants and how to landscape your yard. Or maybe you were interested in marine life or outer space, but you never had time to study the solar system. Some of you may have been interested in astronomy or the study of fossils. How many of you wanted to learn how to play the piano but didn't have the opportunity?

The physical dexterity required to learn an instrument, as well as mental practice, will stimulate your mind much more than you ever thought. When I turned 69, I decided to learn the piano. The piano is a very difficult instrument to master, and usually you must start young to become a proficient pianist. Many musicians and conductors stay mentally sharp well into their old age.

I took online courses and eventually found a jazz pianist that was willing to take me on as a student. My goal was to learn piano theory without reading sheet music and to develop muscle memory. I wanted to be able to create my own songs and play by ear. By practicing for an hour or more a day, my abilities rapidly improved to where I could just make up songs as I went along. As time moves on, and some of my friends fade away, I will be able to challenge myself and entertain others on the piano by learning new songs through memorization. Sometimes I just develop a musical theme based on my mood, and play that theme for a long time.

Why not give yourself every advantage that you can to keep that brain sharp? The Happy Things to do in Healthy Aging" chapter is a good reference for new ideas. It is never too late.

I have many patients who learned how to use the computer at an older age. They took evening courses at senior centers on how to use the computer, just like my 92-year-old sister did. They became involved in online discussion groups on subjects that interested them and opened their entire world through exploration and fascination. You, too, can become involved through the internet and discover things you never dreamed of. All you need to do is type any word or phrase about any subject in one or more search engines and you will find more web sites than you can read about.

(Do not divulge any personal information or financial information on any unsecured or unfamiliar sites. Or, if you receive urgent notices in your email, call the institution yourself with the phone number you have for them in your records, and not the one on the

notice. Do not click on unknown links, many links may look legitimate but will redirect you to scam web sites – there are a lot of worldwide scam artists waiting to take your money.)

On my world cruise I met a couple that had been married only 5 months, she was 78 and he was 79, they had lived together and decided to get married. After their spouses died, they became lonely and decided to do something about it. Their computer skills allowed them to meet each other on a senior dating site. His hook was standing in front of the Panama Canal in the photo and she asked, "Is that the Panama Canal?" Travel became a common denominator for them. They even co-wrote a book together about how seniors can meet each other online, the safety precautions to take, how to find a compatible new partner and develop a new life.

You know, a lot of people travel when they get older. They go to different locations. How about getting all the information you possibly can about a particular place you might want to visit. If you visit many different places, you will find out about their ancient histories, and the turbulent times they went through from conquests, rebuilding, to cultural attitudes, their clothes, and the type of food they cook. You can really get carried away in ancient civilizations. Also research how safe the area is and what parts of a city to avoid. On my previous transatlantic cruises, many of the people I talked to were in their 70s and some in their 80's. They were sharp and fascinating to talk to. On one of the cruises, I ended up teaching ballroom dance classes because the instructors missed the ship. There were people in their 60's to late 70's learning ballroom dancing and loving it. We switched partners every couple of minutes, and everyone was laughing and having a good time.

In my RV travels through the Maritime Provinces in Canada, I met a lady that was in her mid-sixties that gave away all her stuff, rented her house out in northern California, and decided to travel to see the world. She said, "What am I going to do? Do the same things I've been doing over and over?" She decided that the variety of experiences in different regions of the USA and Canada would be very good for her spirit and mental wellbeing, and she was right. She told me that now she could think about her daily existence, where she is going to go in her RV, where she would stay, how to navigate different cities, explore what there was to see there, etc. Just like the rats in their stimulating environments with new things being added, her mind was constantly being stimulated by the new places she visited, and the novel environments she explored. To keep her company in her RV she bought a small terrier dog that became a perfect travel companion. She spends her evenings reading or working part time in her graphic design business. When she gets to an area that she likes, she stays there a few weeks to get a feel for the area and participates in local activities.

This world is a very large place. It's much larger than that TV or cell phone screen in front of you, trying to sell you something or trying to influence your thoughts. Those nonstop commercials are turning you into a zombie, programming you to purchase anything that has been put into your mind. Do you know that it takes seeing something 14 times in an advertisement before you act on that product? It used to be just 7 times. That's why there are commercials everywhere now, from your smart phone to your gas station pump. Now, with Artificial Intelligence (AI), they will be able to slowly program you to think a certain way, or create a need for a certain product. It's all very subtle, and you will not be aware of what is happening to you. AI knows how to subtly influence you bit by bit till its programmer's desired goal is met. In the end are you still you? Or are you a product of AI programming. Just turn off that TV, stop reading news feed blurbs on your smart phone and enjoy life.

Once again the saying, **"Garbage in, garbage out"** applies here. Try to recognize how much garbage you read in the news, **on your smart phone, in ads, and headlines every single day. They dupe you by saying "click here to continue the story." That click saves your IP address for similar stories to keep you engaged in their content. AI is developing a profile on your likes.**

In the media, most of what you hear about is negative events. Is that healthy for your mind? What about the Optimists' creed I spoke of, or the positive attitude that is essential for the healthy mind. You poison yourself by filling your mind with negative information that is constantly bombarding you through the media. Put that aside. Or, if you are going to do it, use it for specific purposes that are mentally and intellectually stimulating. Check your phone to see how many minutes or hours a day you waste reading those teaser ads and stories.

You can stimulate your mind in thousands of ways, but you need to be creative. If you lack creativity, go to a library reference section, or even on the internet, and start looking up different topics. Look in the occupational handbook for all different types of occupations. For a long time, I have been interested in sailing, boating, scuba diving, and marine life. I spent a great deal of time learning everything I possibly could about those topics. Once I learned them, I moved onto another subject about which I knew very little and tried to educate myself on it.

When I retired, I went back to a local college and learned how to program and develop a website. I learned all the ins and outs of websites, HTML programing, and design. It was another area of my mind that was not developed, and I forced myself to learn new things.

You should be doing the same thing, constantly adding data to your memory banks, constantly increasing the RAM inside your brain. By increasing the RAM, you will increase your processing speed, and you will be able to make connections and rational thought processes quicker. (Jessie, at 94 years old, even knew the names of the USA president and the Canadian Prime Minister.)

Throw in a good attitude and a loving heart and you will have a winning combination for the happy mind. By constantly stimulating your mind you are protecting your neurons.

You keep your neurons from atrophying when you use them. You are also producing something called a brain-derived growth factor. You see, this growth factor, just like growth hormone, is produced by the brain, and it is stimulated by mental activity, which nurtures your dendrites and causes them to sprout, but you must have the stimulus.

It's kind of like sexual attraction. You need a stimulus to develop your interest, the looks, the smell, the ambience, the attractiveness of the other person, the conversation, etc. You also need a stimulus for brain growth factor, arousal, which is a challenging and stimulating mental environment. That stimulus gets the growth factor aroused and says, "Hey, I'm turned on. Let's make some more brain cells. Let's get some more endorphins pumping in here so that I feel great." It's a chain reaction, just like the motto, "smile awhile and soon the smile gets more smiles." The brain likes it. If the brain is happy, you are happy because you remember things, you feel invigorated, you have lots of energy, and you have lots of stamina. It all starts in the mind. You must jump start it by stimulating your mind.

Once you've learned something about one subject or discipline, such as math, archeology, playing a musical instrument or learning a language, go to a totally different area of interest and develop that as well, because the brain deteriorates selectively. It loses brain fiber in areas that are not being used, in reference to the Use It or Lose It Principle.

If you only use a small portion of your brain to do a few things, the other parts of your brain will wither. Older people lose brain mass because they are not learning new things. It's just like your muscles or your bones when they're not used. What happens if you put your arm in a cast for a few months and don't use it? The muscles atrophy and the arm become weaker. You must constantly use muscles and bones to keep them healthy. The same goes for your brain.

The reason I advocate for changing topics is that a different topic and a different field of interest will in effect buttress those areas that are lacking in stimulation. We know, through EEG and Pet Scans that specific areas of the brain light up when new thoughts and activities are created.

Maybe you will need to go out each week and do a different activity or something different every day of the week. Wouldn't that be interesting? Just like they did with those rats, when they changed their environment every single day, or the lady traveling in her motor home. You could also join meetup groups on the internet having different fields of interest.

People are not designed to live in a retirement complex with nothing but old people sitting around in chairs not talking to each other. **Humans are designed to live in environments made up of a large variety of stimuli and be socially engaged either through family or a network of friends**. Old people living with young children, old people living with pets, old people going out to different environments (not just the mall), playing games, traveling, living life to the fullest.

The thing that is wrong with growing old gracefully is that you become the old/old. You want to be the young/old, the healthy 100-year-olds. You want your biological age to be younger than your chronological age.

For those who just sit around playing Scrabble, Pinochle or Mahjong with their friends, the only part of their brain that will stay developed is the Scrabble or Mahjong part. What about listening to Beethoven or seeing that Monet painting in the museum? Do you know the artwork or the different eras they come from? Do you know the different styles of the artists? How about the latest theories of Gestalt therapy, psychological therapy, new thoughts on substance abuse, eating disorders, or the local dance company's interpretation of Swan Lake? Or, going to a swing dance with all ages dancing? Myrna, an 85-year-old lady friend, goes swing dancing weekly and all her new friends are younger. Her older friends died so she replaced them with younger friends that now call her periodically to do things with them.

You can also to figure out how to get the most out of all the programs you have on your computer by reading those program manuals, or learn to data mine resources on the internet. Talk about mental stimulation; that would certainly get your brain going and possibly allow you to make better investments and lifestyle decisions.

You can do it.

All it takes is the will to do it, the will to live life to its fullest, the will to be a young/old instead of an old/old. The baby boomers do not want to get old. They want to stay physically and mentally active. They want to continue to have fun and live life to their fullest. The only way to do it is to continue stimulating and using your mind in all its aspects. Prevent the atrophy that happens with age. Promote an inspiring environment. Live in an invigorating environment.

Do not live in an old person's place. Live in a place populated with people of all ages, different ideas, different stimuli, and different lifestyles. Do you realize that old farts who do nothing, who live in deed-restricted communities, looking for deed violations, thinking of only themselves, are aging their brains prematurely because they're not open to new ideas? They are not accepting other lifestyles, nor even accepting assorted colors of houses. How dull can you be?

That is the kind of stuff that ages you, ladies and gentlemen, lack of acceptance and lack of diversity. Always the same old/same old makes you the same old, boring, and old. You want to live among artists. You want to live among creative people of all ages. You want to live in an environment that is stimulating and uplifting, with as little stress as possible, and as little discord as possible.

Live and let live. Enjoy life. Accept diversity among others. Learn from that diversity. Don't complain (the grumpy old man or lady syndrome). Be happy. Look at the positive aspect of everything you see. Look at the beauty in the sky, join an astronomy or bird watching club. Have you ever thought about the flight patterns of birds, or why they migrate? How about the courtship patterns of the Osprey bird? I spoke of this a little when discussing the pineal gland in my Happy Life Healthy Aging book. If you do not like Ospreys pick a famous painter or composer and compare their style to another artist, or better yet take a drawing class.

Some of you may be saying, "Come on, this is getting a little far-fetched." Well, it isn't. I am trying to get you to stimulate your mind in as many ways as possible in order to have that longevity mind. I want you to pay attention to the environment around you. Give your brain a jump-start. Change your daily routine. Expose yourself to an unfamiliar environment daily. Do different things every day and not the same routine all the time. This is why I like cruising on ships, different locations, environments, enrichment lectures and nightly entertainment.

On another book's first re-write trip I had no set travel plans. I made things up as I went along, visited people and places that gave me further insight into how to improve my old book "Seven Secrets of Anti-Aging", which later turned into "Happy Life Healthy Aging". In Prince Edward Island, Canada, I met a retired couple from Germany traveling in their RV. They had shipped their small motor home and in five months traveled over 33,000 kilometers (20,000 miles). They went across Canada all the way to Anchorage Alaska and back. They will ship their RV back to Germany because they still enjoyed exploring Europe as well. The couple were parked next to me. I was curious about their German license plate and started talking to them. Throughout the day the lady was constantly reading something.

For this book, I decided to simplify the scientific aspect and observe how people aged on a 133 day world cruise. A world cruise is the perfect environment to observe an older population in their various stages of physical and mental aging.

"Okay, okay," you say. "I've had enough data. Now tell me what to do." Here is a summary.

Read as much as you can about a variety of subjects. Make sure the subjects are diverse, as in the previous examples I highlighted. Perhaps something mathematical or technical. Then change the next subject to psychological or physiological. Get involved in the arts, which are highly brain-stimulating. Be involved in human interactions around young, exciting, different-thinking people. Get outside your comfort zone. Explore the universe just like that German couple was doing. They went outside their comfort zone and started exploring places they had never been to before.

Do you remember how I told you to make a list of things you have always been interested in but never had time to pursue? Well, when are you going to make the time?

The time is now. Make that list. Make it as long as possible because the longer the list, the longer you will have something to look forward to. If you have something new to look forward to every single day of your life, something that is exciting, your mind is going to be excited. The endorphin levels are going to be high. You are going to be full of life. Your quality of life will increase exponentially.

You've heard of the empty nest syndrome. People downsize and sell their homes because they don't need the room anymore. They buy a small condominium or townhouse. Suddenly, they have nothing to do. With the children grown, they have lost their purpose in life. It is no wonder that many divorces also occur in this stage of life.

You must regain that purpose through new experiences, new interests, and new enthusiasm. That is going to keep your mind healthy and young. Coupled with physical activity, this will stimulate those brain growth factors, protect you from free radical damage, sprout those new neurons to produce new dendrites and increase the connectors in your brain. But you need to do it. No matter what I say, unless you get out there and do it, your mind will not stay young. Did you know that fifty percent of brain cells are already gone when someone finally gets diagnosed with Alzheimer's disease? You want to constantly stimulate that mind to grow new cells as well as to have a greater reserve of cells to function with.

Throughout this book, I speak about the natural approaches towards longevity. Yes, there are different drugs and chemicals that artificially try to stimulate your mind, the problem is, I don't know what else they may be doing to you. You may be destroying yourself in the long run. Any benefits from them are short lived.

Stick to the natural approaches. Stimulate your mind and get involved emotionally through loving your neighbor, your spouse. Do charitable deeds, which will bring further happiness to the environment around you.

What about playtime? I believe playtime is just as important as mental stimulation for a healthy mind. It stimulates the limbic system, the emotional system, the gut feeling you get of pure pleasure when you do something fun.

What you want to achieve are positive emotions, like cheerfulness, overall happiness, and the joy of living. Much of that comes from doing fun things, both individually and in group activities.

Social interaction has recently been shown to be one of the most important components of healthy aging. In

"Aging Well" a book written by George E. Vaillant, MD, the long-term study of Adult Development was examined. In various studies, such as the Harvard University Study of Adult Development or the Inner-City Study, analyses were made to determine how well people aged throughout their entire life. These long-term 50-year studies of individuals, no matter their education or socioeconomic status, showed that those who stayed socially engaged did much better in their physical and mental health than those that became isolationists. They had a happier and more fulfilling retirement.

Social interaction through volunteering, interest groups, dancing, or sport is important because it falls into this limbic, gut-reaction activity level. It applies to this having fun category. Social contact hones your interactive skills. It stimulates you to create new and random thoughts, as well as the inventing of ideas. Bantering back and forth is healthy. It gives you an interest and pizzazz. Did you ever wonder why people love to gossip? It gives them an emotional boost. It gets the juices running. Even gossip is an anti-aging technique, so long as it is not destructive.

We must do fun things to stimulate our emotions. We need playtime. Figure out what is fun for you. Make that list of things you have always wanted to do or are interested in. Have you ever thought of making a list of people you want to associate with, or people you wanted to know? I bet you never thought of that, did you?

On my world cruise, I met a Canadian couple that would invite the entertainers to sit at their table. Most of the time, when asked, the entertainers said yes to joining them at their table. They enjoyed getting to know them personally and finding out how they ended up as entertainers on ships.

When you make that list of the type of people you want to hang around with include the interests they have, their activity level, their intellectual level, their educational level, their past life experiences, their attitudes towards life. This is as important to you at your older age as it is to a teenager making younger friends.

You know the old saying, the type of people you hang around with will be the kind of person you will become. Sure, you've told your children to stay away from undesirable people or people who are bad influences. So what about you when you get older? Why don't you follow your own advice? Stay away from people who have bad influences on you, especially from negative people. They'll wear you out and take you down to the dumps with them.

Chronic complainers are chronic complainers. Who wants to hear that? You want to hang around with people who are young in mind and young in spirit, full of life, ideas, and vitality. People who love to have fun. People who are physically active in all types of sports, and especially people who stay mentally active. You may even choose friends who have different levels of activity just so you are exposed to different stimuli. You choose your friends. After all, you have free will. You don't need to be stuck with the same people repeatedly.

You're probably asking, "How do you select people as friends? How do you get out of this rut of doing the same thing with the same people?" You do it by taking charge of your actions.

Go through that list of things you always wanted to do or things you may possibly be interested in. Look for clubs, internet meetup groups and organizations that do those things. Join those clubs or organizations, be it an antique car group, a Porsche rally group, a bicycle group, or the local Writer's Guild. Find out where these organizations are, go to their meetings, meet the people, find the people you like, and start doing things with them. It's a lot easier than you think. At the Villages, an active central Florida retirement community with 140,000 people and growing, there are over 3,000 social and lifestyle clubs. Of course, you need to be mobile to do that, to get ideas look at the physical activity section of this book.

It is of utmost importance to maintain physical activity in order to preserve joint stability, prevent aches and pains, and in turn allow you to do a variety of things. Everything is a cascade of events. You must go from point A to get to point B, point B to get to point C. You can't skip things just by taking a magic pill. You've got to put effort into your anti-aging program. You put effort into building your life, now put effort into maintaining your life.

At the library in St Johns Memorial University in Newfoundland Canada, I met a doctor writing a thesis. She complained to me that her patients expect her to just give them a pill to fix everything and not take responsibility for their health. That does not work, the universe does not work that way. You must do preventive maintenance on everything in this world including your mind and your body.

Your longevity program will become a lot of fun, especially if you choose those things that really interest you. You will have fascinating friends, an interesting lifestyle, and many things to be involved in. Your time will be so full you will wonder how you ever had time to work before. You will have an action-packed, fun-filled retirement; or should I say, a new vocation, which is anti-aging fun.

Let's just change the topic slightly and talk about staying partially active during your career to prevent aging. You have seen people have midlife crises, quitting what they're doing in their forties or fifties and taking on a totally different occupation. This happens because people get bored, their work becomes unstimulating, or they have always had an interest in something else and feel they are now financially capable of pursuing that interest.

Your healthy aging mind program could also involve staying active in your career. If you have a job that is mentally stimulating and interesting, why quit? Stay in that job or career on a part-time basis, but make sure you are doing something you enjoy doing. It's also great for your pocketbook because you won't have to dip into your retirement savings all the time. If you have plenty of money, give the extra money away to charity or provide a scholarship for a needy child who is mentally gifted and cannot afford the tuition for university.

There is a lot of good you can do in society. By volunteering your expertise or your professional time you are helping society as a whole and giving back. Life is too short to be miserable working at a job you don't enjoy. It is of utmost importance that you get a boost out of what you do for a living. You need to feel you really like doing your job. I remember going through my practice. Yes, there are ups and downs, there will be certain people you don't care to see because they are downers, but, overall, I remember many times going into my practice saying, "Boy, I really love what I'm doing, this is so much fun."

After a while, during retirement, you get tired of playing golf or deep-sea fishing. Then, you say to yourself, "What else is there to do?" If you pace yourself in a progressive longevity program, make your list of things you want to do, keep yourself mentally active, learn new things, and stay physically active, your mind and your body should stay young.

I figured that for me it was better to work on a part-time basis in my profession for a while and then retire after a few years when newer interests developed. Since I love medicine, I stay active in my specialty of physical medicine and rehabilitation through volunteering at a free clinic. I also go to weekly continuing medical education seminars in my area to stay current in medicine.

I especially liked my chelation/nutritional patients because those people were older and so full of life. Many of the ideas I am telling you in this book I learned from observing my successful older patients who came to me to stay young and maintain their health.

I interviewed them extensively. My medical history questionnaire was very thorough. It covered everything: How many children they had, how many spouses, whether or not they're happy, if they've had psychiatric treatment, any health ailments, medical treatments, medications, supplements, hobbies, what they did in their careers and their lives. By having such extensive data on older people, I was able to observe what worked and what didn't.

What I am informing you of in this book are things that work, especially the mental attitudes that people have towards their life, and how they planned things to get to where they are now.

Successful longevity doesn't happen spontaneously. People who are successful in older age plan their success all along by following anti-aging principles. By following my patients, the randomness of insights became less random and more consistent. A little research here, a little research there. Comments here and there. An attitude here and an attitude there. From that, you can get a picture of how people do best as they age. You get a picture of how people stay physically active and disease-free as they age. You get a picture of how people stay mentally clear and involved in life as they age. You get a blueprint for a darn good longevity program that is do-able.

What I am describing is a compilation of current research and observation; things you can do. Yes, you have genes that can affect your outcome to a certain extent. But even if you do have genes stacked against you, you can modify genetic activity through what you do. The new science of epigenetics studies how environment and behavior modify genes. Just as I have seen physical activity studies based on identical twins, I know the same thing is true in all other aspects of healthy aging.

I know that people can will themselves into living longer, will themselves to be happy, and will themselves to modify their disease processes.

The mind is powerful. It can be stimulated to produce the right chemicals, fabricate a happy environment for the cells, and generate growth and sprouting of new cells. Give it adequate oxygenation through increased circulation and physical activity, give it a variety of mental stimulation and it will be very happy, rewarding you with a long, prosperous, and happy life.

Even if you have a neurodegenerative disease where you cannot be as mobile as you want, push yourself. Use rehabilitative exercises to resurface your joints, to strengthen your muscles and bones. Get back on track, but also keep your mind going. Keep it interested. Keep it diverse. Learn new things. Continue doing the fun things you used to love to do. Associate with fun-loving, interesting people, then you will have a blast into your silver years.

If you are in a stressful environment, get out of it. Life is too short to put up with a stressful environment. You have decision-making abilities. It is your life you are playing with. Do something about it.

Surround yourself with stress-free people, stress-free environments, and a fun-filled mentally stimulating environment. Change your activity every day. Have new stimuli every day. Make a list for 365 days of the year of what you are going to do and go through that list and follow through. If that's too long, make a thirty-day list, or even a seven-day list. Just do it.

Set new goals for yourself. Write down what you want to do every month, every year, and pursue those goals. The important part is that you write those goals down, write those lists down, and check them off as you do them. Be methodical. This way, you will stimulate every single part of your brain. You know, this whole program is free. Libraries don't cost much. All you need is a pair of walking shoes and a desire to stay young. What you put into your mind is just as important as what you put into your mouth. Garbage in is garbage out like on the internet.

If you are under a tremendous amount of stress or negative emotions, your body is going to react to it. You will have decreased resistance. You're going to get more illnesses.

There were studies done in Britain in which people were exposed to a cold virus. The ones under the highest stress had the highest chances of catching a cold. Stress reduces the power of your immune system to protect itself and you are then much more susceptible to any disease process that comes along. As I mentioned in the introduction, stress has been linked to just about every disease of our modern society, from cancer to heart disease to high blood pressure, stroke, skin condition, allergies, you name it, and they can be stress-induced.

Dr. Hans Selye, a Hungarian-Canadian endocrinologist, did an excellent job in his book, "The Stress of Life", in pointing out how prolonged stress can gradually destroy our immune system. It has to do with the cortisol level, which, when unchecked, gradually reduces our immunity and slowly kills us.

You need to counteract stressful situations by getting out of them. Eliminate anything in your life that prevents you from having happy thoughts and peace of mind. You are not a victim of circumstance. You can always change the circumstances around you. Sometimes a small change can make a big difference to your peace of mind. You are in charge.

You can even change your inner thought processes by visualizing happier times in your life, which will put you in a relaxed state and help boost your immune system. Rent funny movies and watch them to reduce your stress level. Laughter therapy has been shown to be successful in beating even the greatest diseases. Of course, one of the best ways to reduce stress is to engage in play time, doing things that you love to do, be it dancing, bicycling, bird watching, or any activity that gives you great physical pleasure. A friend, the CEO of a corporation with his own private jet, removed himself from the stress. He just quit. All his friends were six feet under. He was able to break free of the stressful situation, quit his job and live a happy, stress-free existence sailing in Florida.

He changed his destiny, happily lived a long time, and so can you. Put some time and thought into it. What can you do to change your environment, reduce your stress load, and stimulate your mind? I have always thought the work week was a little screwed up. We work five days a week and have two days off.

How about if we turn it around by working two days a week and have five days off? Wouldn't that be a wonderful situation to be in? We work part-time and play most of the time. The play time would certainly reduce your stress level, allowing you to pursue all kinds of interests, stimulating different areas of the brain that needed a tune up to stay young. Maintaining part-time work would give you enough money so you would not have to dig into your savings as much, as well as keep you mentally and physically involved in a job you used to enjoy, making you feel productive in the workforce and useful to the rest of society. When we feel needed and appreciated, we will get a lot more out of the job environment, and we will contribute a lot more toward that job environment. The job environment can also be a volunteer position in which you use your past skills to teach others to become successful in those skills.

Remember, happy thoughts are essential toward a successful longevity program. Mental stimulation is essential in healthy aging. Stress reduction is essential for healthy longevity as well as physical activity.

Stress to your body is like toxins in your food. Toxins poison you slowly. Stress poisons your mind and slowly destroys your body also.

Happy thoughts, mental stimulation, social engagement and peace of mind are the magic pills that keep you healthy. **A healthy aging mind is a happy mind. It is a stress-free mind. It is a stimulated mind**. It is an inquisitive mind. It is a mind that loves to have social interaction, a mind that wants to continually learn new things, a mind that is continually developing, and a mind that is happy. **Whatever the mind can conceive, it can achieve.** If you truly want a longevity program that keeps you young, well into your nineties and over a hundred, the time to start action is now. **You can do it.** Only you can do it.

The other alternatives are not very pleasing. You do not want to reserve that bed in the nursing home when you're seventy. You don't want to reserve that bed at all. You want to stay active until you drop dead at 105.

CHAPTER 4

The Physical Activity Drug

The most important and cheapest designer drug you can take is **physical activity**. There is no other medication that does as much for you pharmacologically, physiologically and structurally than being physically active. While food is the building block of your body, exercise is the engine. Exercise keeps everything lubricated and working, preventing a host of debilitating conditions that keep you from enjoying the rest of your life.

Physical activity, along with caloric restrictions, requires the greatest amount of self-control and self-discipline. Since I am a specialist in orthopedic medicine and rehabilitation, this is a topic dear to my heart. I have produced twenty-eight specific rehabilitative exercise videos (VCR exercises) to restore joint mobility and strengthen surrounding muscles.

I also lectured to international physicians interested in integrative medicine at the anti-aging course at the American College for Advancement of Medicine (ACAM). **Most of these physicians did not fully realize the importance of physical activity in longevity.** During my lecture, I asked everyone to stand in place and walk for the entire hour. I tried to maintain a fairly steady pace and I counted out the cadence for the doctors to walk in place. Periodically during my lecture, I looked out to the audience to see how they were doing. I urged them on to keep up the pace.

After fifteen minutes, and even more so after thirty minutes, a percentage of my audience stopped exercising or greatly slowed down. Mind you, these are physicians interested in anti-aging. That's why they're taking the course. How can doctors, proponents to be pioneers in integrative medicine and preventative medicine, be in such poor shape? Have they merely substituted pill pushing from big, mega-billion-dollar drug companies to vitamin pushing, or are they truly serious in making a change in themselves and their patients.

I'm happy to say there were many in the audience who were vigorous in their exercise efforts, some even jumping up and down from one leg to the other, raising their knees high to get the full benefit of the exercise. They continue that marathon effort throughout the entire hour. Obviously there are some physicians who want to set good examples for their patients. Those are the doctors you want to go see.

We live in a society of instant fixes. We want everything now. We want youth now. We want fun now. We want money now. We want things now on credit. We want self-gratification and self-indulgence now. Well, I hate to break the bad news to you, your body just does not work that way.

You can't cheat nature. The rules of nature have been laid down over millions of years. Genes have mutated multiple times in over one hundred thousand years, to maximize our species survival. You must be physically active to maintain joint function, muscle tone, mental acuity, hormonal function, and crucial metabolic pathways such as sugar transfer from our blood to our cells. **Exercise activates SIRT genes.** These genes are involved in multiple biological processes, including **DNA repair, cellular energy and slowing down the aging process**.

Movement is life. Every atom in the universe has movement. Even steel atoms have movement. The cesium 131 atom has 9 billion oscillations/second, this resonant frequency determines the time of a second on the Atomic Clock at the National Standards Laboratory. Nerve and muscle cells have movements. A brain wave pattern involves movements. Our thoughts involve movements that transfer electro-chemical messages from one cell to another. The basic law of motion is universal. **Without movement, there is death.**

One of the great baseball players of the twentieth century thought that life was like a bar of soap. You gradually wear it out until there is nothing left. In his time frame, it made sense. But, in the twenty-first century, it does not make sense because we know a lot more about human physiology. We know a lot more about nerve transmission and mental acuity. We know you can take a feeble, frail, nursing home patient in his nineties and within two months, rehabilitate his muscle strength and increase it by 174%. We know that. The baseball player didn't.

No matter how old you are, you can always improve your muscular performance significantly. Muscle cells do not just wear away like a bar of soap. They can be rebuilt, re-toned, strengthened. Your muscular strength and tone are directly related to your ability to be active when you are older. Why did the eighty-eight-year-old ball player at the Kids 'n Kubs baseball field walk with a brisk pace, pick up a bat, and walk back to the dugout just like a forty year old? Because he maintained his muscle tone and activity level. He was **continuously active** when he got older. In other words, he put in effort.

You have got to plan ahead. **What you put in is exactly what you get out. There are no shortcuts.** I know how hard it is to get out there and exercise three times a week. But I'll help you. At the end of this chapter, I'll give you **the Lenhart Physical Activity Formula for Anti-Aging**, derived after considerable research and analysis of hundreds of research articles, as well as personal experience through observation of patients and neighbors.

Seventy four percent of the U.S. population is overweight or obese. Probably a greater percentage is inactive. Let's look at those statistics in economic terms. How many hundreds of billions of dollars have been made by the fast food industry to put on those wasted pounds? How many more billions were made by the biochemical industry to invent and process food so that it stays fresh forever, looks good, and tastes good? These chemists make a lot of money inventing chemicals to artificially fertilize the soil and kill all the pests in it, chemicals to grow food rapidly, create pest resistant plants and produce chemicals to preserve food and maintain its texture. They also genetically modified our food. As a matter of fact, they are engineering pesticides to be built into the plants so spraying of crops will not be necessary. Soon they will produce genetically altered beef and chicken. The animals will grow faster and slaughterhouses will become more profitable.
Let's continue the economic aspect of your behavior further. **Due to your poor lifestyle habits, the medical industry will get larger and larger**.

Baby boomers grew up on fast food, additives, chemicals, comfortable couches, easy chairs, sucrose sweetened sodas and high-sugar munchies. As they age, drug companies and some hospitals will make lots of money because those Boomers will need continual medical care.

Drug companies will compete at breakneck speed to create new magic pills to fight these western diseases we have because of our poor lifestyles. They will also try to create pills where we do not have to exercise at all.

Governments will be near bankruptcy because of the high costs of Medicare and Medicaid and other social programs. In order to supply all the services to those who didn't plan ahead, didn't take care of their bodies, taxes will have to go up and younger people will balk at paying those taxes.

Baby boomers are retiring at the rate of ten thousand a day. That is a huge stressor on our health care system and something has to give. Less coverage? More co-pay? Use your imagination how the government will react to this extra burden on the system. They may even set age or disease based treatment quotas, who knows?

If you don't use it, you lose it.

If you sit back, relax, and do not put any effort into a preventive anti-aging health care program, you will suffer the consequences in the later stages of life.

Increasing your physical activity is the absolute cheapest, most efficient, most effective way to increase your chances of prolonging your life substantially, and at the same time, decrease all the diseases that plague us in our older age such as metabolic syndrome. Physical activity done on a consistent, regular basis is, just by itself, the best healthy aging treatment available even without adding all the other possibilities mentioned in this book. The more ideas in this book you incorporate, the greater your odds for a healthier, disease-free, mentally alert retirement.

About thirty seven years ago, I moved into a neighborhood in which one neighbor was a very elderly gentleman; at least, he looked very elderly. He was seventy-three-years-old, frail, pale, and walked real slow. I saw him start to go on short walks up and down the block on a daily basis. Eventually he started bike riding and increased his distance progressively.

Over the years as I watched this gentleman, I saw this old, frail person turn into a vigorous, strong, youthful individual. By the time he was eighty-five, he was walking at about a 3.5 mph pace in the morning and evening. If you saw him from the rear, not knowing how old he was, you would swear that he walked and looked like a forty-year-old. His legs had good muscle tone. He has a spring to his walk. He walked deliberately with a cadence and arm swing that one sees in younger people. He was physiologically young and chronologically old.

Before this gentleman started his walking program, he was very, very ill and near death. The persistent, continuous physical activity that he made himself do, not only caused him to recover, but it also caused him to grow biologically younger. It increased his stamina and kept him from developing many age-related diseases.

One day I asked him what else he did to keep himself so young and fit and he said he lifted weights on a regular basis to keep up his muscle tone.

I have since observed other individuals following a similar protocol of continued physical activity who were able to stay young well into their eighties and nineties.

Bruce, the 87 year old head of our Sunday Bladers roller blading and bicycle group, is one of them. He does the Monday, Thursday and Sunday skates every week on his bicycle. He makes the schedule, takes photos and writes a blog after each skate.

Zumba is one of the best complex movement aerobic exercises that helps grow your brain along with dancing. Zumba involves movement of the arms, hands, legs, torso and feet all at the same time. It is different from step aerobics because you are also patterning your arms and hands. This movement is synchronized to music and a lot harder to do than it looks. In Alzheimer's disease or Parkinson's, complex movement training is important for delaying symptoms or possibly stopping them. Complex movements use multiple pathways and provide redundancy. For babies, cross crawl patterning helps develop neuronal pathways. As the baby crawls from one place to another, he or she is growing their brain connectors. They use contralateral limb movement, such as right hand forward and left knee forward to train their neuronal pathways. In Zumba you also perform cross crawl patterns.

In Alzheimer's, Parkinson's or Lewy body disease, which is a form of Parkinson's, you want to have as much residual capacity to rely on as possible, in order to compensate for neuronal decay. You also want to increase your pulse and your brain circulation through aerobic activity.

Robert, a physician friend of mine, who was once the hospital chief of staff, started to develop Parkinson's disease in his early 80s. He immediately started a comprehensive exercise program, because he knew that exercise was effective in delaying Parkinson's.

People that go from simple forgetfulness, such as where did I put my keys or parked my car to noticeable Alzheimer's disease, have decreased brain circulation. Zumba gives you many of the same benefits as dancing. Aerobic activity, music therapy, balance, bone strengthening, ligament toning and coordination. You can watch Zumba on line or better yet attend Zumba classes. When you finish a half hour Zumba session you are sweating and feel good about yourself.

Dancing is another excellent means of maintaining physical activity into old age. I noticed this with my uncle who went ballroom dancing twice a week. He died in his nineties. He did not even follow any other longevity programs, as outlined in this book. All he did was increase his physical activity by dancing twice a week well into old age.

Through my ballroom and swing dance experiences, I have been able to observe very healthy retires who are my dance partners. Some of those ladies are proud to tell me that they are 85 or 87 years old and that dancing keeps them going. After several years of observing how alert and fit these dancers were, I decided to write **"Dance to Live"**. The book spells out all of the health, longevity and social benefits of dancing. You will be surprised what dancing does for your balance, muscle strength, endurance, social interaction, coordination, your bones and your mind. Dancing allows older widows and widowers to touch someone in a safe environment. Touch is very important for our wellbeing. Babies need touch in order to thrive.

Why is maintaining physical activity so important? It is important because it regulates your hormones, it preserves and strengthens your muscles, joints, ligaments, tendons, and bones. At the same time, it conditions your cardiovascular system and increases waste elimination. By pumping your muscles, you are forcing excretion of waste products that have accumulated. Increased cardiovascular stress due to the exercise conditions and strengthens your heart.

You may be asking at this time, "What does exercise have to do with conditioning your bones." To tell you the truth, most doctors don't know either. Only the physicians who have studied radiology realize there is direct correlation of both growth and strength, which is directly proportional to the stress placed on the bone.

There is a law in radiology and bone growth called the **Wolff's Law**, stating that the bone will directly remodel itself based upon the force applied to it. In other words, putting it in laymen's terminology, **the bone gets stronger only if it is stressed**. If you do not put stress on the bone, it becomes soft, weak, brittle, and subject to breaks.

What is one of the most common disabilities that occurs to older individuals? Hip fractures and other bone fractures. When people age, they don't stress their bones enough to make them strong. Any type of small trauma can cause the bone to break. When the bones break, people become immobilized. Then begins a downward cycle.

Immobility leads to muscle wasting. Muscle wasting leads to incapacitation. Incapacitation leads to further degeneration, loss of the ability to perform activities of daily living, and eventually, death. How many people have you known who broke bones at an elderly age, never recovered, and rapidly thereafter, ended up dying? ICU patients can lose 20% of their muscle mass in 10 days.

Did you know that one week of bed rest causes you to lose ten percent of your muscle mass? Bed rest also induces **total body insulin resistance**.

Every subsequent week of bed rest causes you to lose another ten percent of the residual muscle mass. It does not take a mental genius to figure out how weak you can become in a very short period of time by not moving or stressing your muscles. The greatest amount of muscle strength loss occurs in the early stages of bed rest.

If you don't believe me, look at the astronauts. What happens after they return from space missions? Do they have to be helped out of their space vehicles? We've seen it many times. They come out frail, weak, and unsteady on their feet. That's because they didn't have the opportunity to stress their bones and muscles adequately enough in space.

It all goes back to the same rule. **If you don't use it, you lose it** ..... Rapidly.

Let's get back to the bed rest patients. How long do you think it would take for them to regain their muscle mass? If they lose ten percent of their muscle mass with one week of bed rest? In order to regain that, it would take maximum contraction of the muscles on a daily basis for one week to regain only ten percent of the muscle mass they lost. Now, they have to do this for every muscle group that has been weakened. That's a heck of a lot of work to regain ten percent.

Think of it: If you lose twenty percent or more of your muscle mass due to bed rest, but you can regain only ten percent of your muscle mass at maximum work of every muscle group. That doesn't seem fair does it, but that's the way biology works.

You must continue to use your muscles, ligaments, and tendons and put stress on your bones to maintain function and prevent disability.

If you look at the Kids 'n Kubs 1998 world champion baseball team in St. Petersburg, whose members were all over eighty, you'll see that they have maintained a joyful, physical-activity-filled retirement. They have continuously moved their bodies, stressed their joints, ligaments, and tendons and constantly maintained muscle tone, which preserved the joints, bones, and overall health.

Going back to my **rehabilitation literature**, let's go over what happens to your body with inactivity. Let's see how many diseases you will recognize simply due to immobility. By explaining to you the **body's responses to immobility**, you will be able to determine the beneficial effect of physical activity almost immediately because the effects of immobility and inactivity are just about the same as the effects of aging.

Your **central nervous system**, which is the electrical system for your body, reacts to immobilization by decreasing your sensations. It decreases your ability to move. Your motions change, as well as your behavior, and you start to lose intellectual ability. In other words, **you cannot think as clearly**.

Your **muscular system**, which makes all your bones move and gives you propulsion, allows you to stand, breathe, sit, and walk, not only loses up to twenty percent of its initial strength during one week of bed rest, but with immobilization, the **endurance decreases, the muscles atrophy, and you lose coordination.**

What about your **bones**? I mentioned before that bones react to the stresses placed upon them. With immobilization, you get osteoporosis. You've heard of that. **Osteoporosis is thinning of the bone, which leads to fractures, which leads to disability, which eventually leads to death.**

You also get **fibrosis**. This means you get scar tissues forming at your joints causing them to eventually fuse so you cannot move. Well, that's a bummer. **If you can't move, you're in a dying state because the reverse of dying is movement.**

Then there's your **cardiovascular system**, your heart and circulation. With immobility, you get increased heart rate. You get **low blood pressure** when you stand up or sit up, causing you to pass out. You also get blood clots. **Blood clots lead to inability to breathe and suffocation, or, if they go to the brain, you get a stroke.**

All that happens because you are not moving. You also get what is called a decreased cardiac reserve. The heart just cannot pump as well to get the blood to the vital organs and muscles.

What about your breathing? What happens to your breathing if you get immobilized? Well, **you can't breathe as well**. You cannot take in as much air because of what is known as a restrictive impairment. You're not getting as much oxygen because there is less oxygen going across your membranes and you need oxygen to live. One of the worse things that happens is you **can't cough as much**. So, what's the big deal?

Well, just think about it. We have to cough to get "crud" out of our lungs. If we **accidentally aspirate something** or if we have a cold or if we just have mucous building up in our lungs, we have to be able to cough to move it out. If you cannot cough, you'll get a major infection, and you can die because the lungs fill up with fluid. That increased fluid is a great opportunity for bacteria to set in and **give you pneumonia and fever, which can lead to death**; or worse, a virus gets in there and you get viral pneumonia, which we cannot treat with antibiotics. Unless you have great resistance, which you don't because you are immobilized and not moving, you will most likely die. All because you are not moving, which is something that is preventable for the most part. Unfortunately, it's a downward spiral.

How about **your digestive system**? You lose your appetite and become **constipated**. What about **your kidneys**? You end up **peeing more**. You end up losing some of your sodium, which is very important for your body. You end up **losing calcium**. That explains why you **become osteoporotic**; calcium is taken out of your bone. You end up getting **kidney stones**, which are extremely painful.

What about **your skin**? The skin starts to atrophy. Atrophy is a wearing away or **thinning of the skin** and you end up getting **bed sores**. Bed sores lead to big **ulcers,** which lead to infections it is a really messy situation.

What I have described to you is how the systems in the body break down just by immobilization and inactivity. If you look at older, frail, immobile individuals, you will see the same symptoms I described. **It is a cascade of events. One thing leads to another, to another, until eventually someone dies**.

Let me give you an example, about the "**oldest man in Japan**". He lived in Okinawa, an island that I visited, it is one of the **blue zone** areas in the world where people live for a long time. The island was noted for high nutrient foods, low calorie, restricted diets. He reached 112-years-old. He did agricultural work until he was eighty-five. That means he was doing hard, physical labor to keep his muscles and joints moving. He remained active after he stopped doing farm work. He was a Type A personality, very active mentally and physically. His blood tests were normal. He was able to take care of himself completely until he was 108-years-old when something happened to him and he had to go to a hospital. Well, guess what happened?

Once he got to the hospital, he lost control of his life, his individuality and movements. What happens in a hospital? **Immobilization**. He deteriorated rapidly. **He went from normal to dementia in three years**. This is a good example of what immobility does to you in a very rapid succession, especially if you are older.

What about **immobility of the brain**? The Use It or Lose it principle holds true in all the systems of our body. **Your ability to think clearly and make decisions rapidly is based upon the number of connections you have in your brain called dendrites.** Dendrites are like small branches in an oak tree that fan out and give the tree its shape. Those things talk to each other.

Let's assume you have a dense forest with a lot of these trees with the branches intermingling because they are so tightly packed. The more of these branches you have, the more they are going to intermingle.

Let's say you have a small monkey jumping from one branch to another, and a bigger monkey is chasing him. The more of these little branches intertwined between the trees, the faster he'll be able to run away and make a connection from one tree to the next and elude his predator and the faster will be his forward progress. Therefore, his forward progress will be unimpeded. However, if the trees had few branches and they were further apart, this little monkey would have great difficulty jumping from one tree to the next because there would be fewer branches available for him to grab. His progress would be slowed and he will have a greater chance of being caught by the larger monkey and possibly hurt. **Your brain contracts if you don't have those dendrites.**

Remember the study where rats were placed into a playpen for an hour a day and the objects varied every day? They got to run around and constantly explore new environments. It was a very intellectually stimulating experience for the rats. Plus, a physically charged experience because they had to crawl up and down and around all these objects.

Another group of rats didn't get the exercise and were just placed in a box without a stimulating environment. The rats were then sacrificed and their brains studied.

The brains that were physically and mentally challenged had a large number of connectors (dendrites), like the sprouting branches of a tree, which are evident in very young people because they still have to learn a lot of new things. **The rats not physically and mentally stimulated had considerably fewer connectors**, fewer branches to make connections. That's similar to older people who are not mentally or physically challenged. They have fewer connectors.

You see, people used to think, just like the old bar of soap I mentioned before, that generally, your brain just wears out, deteriorates, and shrinks in size. If you take MRIs of people's brains, you will see atrophy in older individuals. There is a lot more fluid and a lot less gray matter, which is the stuff that does the thinking. However, it does not have to be that way.

There is a group of researchers studying **nuns in Mankato, Minnesota**. They live in a convent and routinely live past their nineties. These nuns were progressive educators, so they donated their brains to science after they died, a noble cause.

It was discovered that the college educated ones lived longer and because the religious order believed that an idle mind is the devil's playground, the nuns constantly did brain exercises crossword puzzles, playing Jeopardy on television, constantly stimulating their minds to think. On autopsy, they found the nuns all had extensive brain dendrite formation at the time of death due to the intellectual stimulation. In other words, they were mentally young. The researchers noted that the ones who stayed mentally active did not suffer from dementia as much as those who didn't.

Newer research is also finding that people who have lost some of their intellectual capacity can regain it by constantly stimulating their brains. They can actually grow new dendrites, not just keep the ones they have, which is a very, very encouraging finding. You can grow intellectually younger just by stressing your brain and making it work, constantly teaching it new things. **It is the old Use It or Lose It philosophy.**

The more I started thinking about this, the more I started thinking about my own life, how I am constantly changing and learning new things. There must be some kind of hidden signal telling me that it is time for me to become intellectually challenged again like writing this book. Once I have learned one topic and used it for a while, I tend to move on to another field of medicine or business or computer science that stimulates my intellect. I go to grand rounds weekly to learn about new advances in medicine. Grand rounds are lectures given in a teaching hospital to further educate physicians and resident physicians. In St Petersburg, Florida, we have two top notch resident teaching hospitals, Bayfront

Medical Center and Johns Hopkins All Children's Hospital that provide me continuous medical education. I also like working on several things at the same time with different intellectually stimulating capacities. **Every different thing you do stimulates a different part of your brain.**

Going back to the Darwinian theory of evolution. Darwin was the guy that did all of his research in the Galapagos Islands off the coast of Ecuador where he discovered different birds developed in different ways and became highly specialized in food gathering and that is why they survived. He had a group of finches that were divergent; they could eat different types of seed and survive in different environments. Others could eat only one type of seed. If that plant became extinct, that species also became extinct.

Your brain works in the same way. It has to have a large variety of stimuli to keep it going and keep it growing. **If you develop only one certain aspect of your brain, the other aspects tend to wither away because they're not being used and not being stimulated.**
You become one-sided and, as your spouse may think, boring. I hate to say this, but people who only talk about one thing, know one thing, work at one thing are not as interesting as people who know a lot about a lot of different things and can hold a variety of conversations on an intellectual level. **A quest for knowledge is one of the most enduring qualities a human can have. That is what differentiates him or her from other mammalian creatures, such as apes.** People that travel a lot, such as on a world cruise, have that quest to explore new cultures and environments. That's how the American Indian ancestors got to America and the Aborigines got to Australia.

Let's summarize this subject by reminding you that **the more connectors you have, the better is your ability to make connections.** It holds true in the business world just as much as **in your brain**. The second part to this is that **intellectual stimulation can cause dendrites to branch out, creating networks of new connections. Use It or Lose It.**

Muscles. What do muscles do? It seems obvious. They hold up your skeleton, protect your organs, and provide movement to the bony part. They **must be used constantly to maintain performance and keep you alive.** If you don't believe me, look at people suffering from muscular dystrophy. You've seen the telethons on television about muscular dystrophy, but you probably never fully realized what that disease does. It slowly destroys your muscles until they wear out. When the muscles wear out, you can't even sit in a wheelchair. After a while, you can't breathe, and you die. That is how important your muscles are. Your heart is a big muscle. According to recent studies done on veterans, **the greater your VO2 max**, the maximum amount of oxygen you can absorb at maximum exertion on a treadmill, **the less chance you have of getting sick.** Cardiovascular and respiratory fitness through exercise is crucial to prolonged healthy living and greater quality of life.

Bones. Bones provide a framework, something to attach things to, such as does your house foundation and outside walls. They provide structure. The bones hold things up. They are attachment points for muscles. They facilitate movements through joints. They allow the joints to move in and out or in circles or whatever different joints in your body do, or talk, as I'm doing right now dictating this book. However, in order for those bones to work properly and not break and fall apart, they need stress to maintain their mineral content and the honeycomb patterns inside the bones that give it strength.

Bones have a honeycomb structure inside them that is kind of a grid like, as used on the Eiffel Tower in Paris, a grid work of iron put together that reinforces one piece to the next and gives it strength. Bones do the same thing. **If you don't stress these bones, if you don't move the bones and constantly use the bones, they lose that grid work and are more prone to fractures.**

When you lose some of that grid work, what happens to the structure? It **weakens.** Just think if you took half the supporting structures out of the Eiffel Tower and a big wind came along. Do you think the Tower would stay standing or do you think it would collapse? The same thing happens to your bones. You have to use them. You have to stress them in order for them to keep on building new bone and creating new supporting structure, called the trabeculae.

Bone is constantly reinforcing itself by any stress put on it to make sure it is the strongest to bear that weight. So, fat people gradually get stronger bones because they have more weight to carry. However, there is a down side to it: The bone joints cannot bear the weight as easily so they wear out.

Bone joints are made of cartilage and cartilage does not rebuild itself as easily as bones do to accommodate the stress placed upon it. Large people develop bad knees and bad joints because too much stress is placed upon those joints. However, if these joints are used constantly and lubricated through motion, there is less chance of them wearing out and greater chance of new layers of cartilage forming over the joint.

There was a study done of a one-year walking program for women. What they found was that over that one year they had an increase of calcium in the top of the hip joint. However, there was no increase in calcium inside the wrist bones. Since women are prone to hip fractures, it showed that **walking increased the strength of their hips**. However, because the stress was only placed upon the hip joints and not the wrists joints. The extra bone deposits were placed where the stress was placed, in the hips.

So, what are the **benefits of healthy bones, muscles, and ligaments**? **You get movement without impediment or disease. You get movement without pain. Isn't that wonderful? You prevent bone damage. You prevent muscular or ligament destruction. You gain power, speed, mobility, freedom, and a greater quality of life. You prevent debilitation and death. Use It or Lose It.**

You may be saying, "That's fine, but I'm ninety. I didn't know about all your data. I didn't read this book till now."

I have good news for you. **A group of ninety-year-olds sitting around in a nursing home with nothing to** do agreed to participate in a strengthening program. They did **eight weeks of high intensity resistance training.** The age group was eighty seven to ninety-six. They trained one muscle group, the quadriceps, which is in the front of your thigh. In just eight weeks, they found increased strength of 174%. One hundred and seventy-four percent in just eight weeks. By strengthening that one muscle group their walking speed increased by 48%. **These were eighty-seven to ninety six year-olds! They were able to rebuild their muscle mass and regain strength by 174%.** To me, that is remarkable. It tells me that Use It or Lose It' does not necessarily mean lose it forever. You can regain it.

Remember, movement is life. If you regain your muscle strength, you regain movement, you regain freedom, and you regain your quality of life.

Take a look at **John Glenn**, the first American to orbit the earth. When he was seventy-seven years old, he returned to space. NASA scientists said he handled the rigors of space every bit as well as astronauts half his age. He suffered no more bone mass loss or muscle loss than the younger astronauts. His heart rate before, during, and after the flight was actually better than the average of twelve younger male astronauts. Isn't that amazing? The message is clear.

At seventy-seven you can do as well as a forty-year-old astronaut.

Glenn walked several miles a day, which I believe is the main reason he did so well. He also did some weight training and ate a balanced diet. Dr. David Williams, director of NASA's Life Science Division and a former shuttle astronaut himself, stated that **Glenn challenged the widespread notion that all seniors are frail individuals.**

John Glenn did just as well as his younger counterparts. He spent four nights in a wired-up sleep suit. He provided seventeen blood samples and wore a small data recorder for twenty-four hours to monitor his heart rate. He also swallowed a capsule holding a radio transmitter and temperature sensor. How much more evidence do you need to see that at just about any age you can become young again through physical activity. **Glenn conditioned himself to the status of a young person. If he lost any functions, he regained them.** An interesting finding was that like all other astronauts, Glenn experienced some balance problems once he returned to earth, but **he recovered just as quickly as the other astronauts**, which surprised the scientists. Many elderly people have difficulty with balance.

You are never too old to start. Exercise improves circulation and cardiovascular life. It also builds and remodels bone and builds new muscle.

There is a study that measured the effects of physical activity and calcium intake on the bone mass of healthy women of different ages. Guess what they found?

If they took calcium alone, it had no effect on their bone mineral density. However, the **people who exercised had a five percent increase in the bone mineral density in the exercised bones.** Remember, I mentioned that you have to put stress on the bone in order for it to grow. However, there was no increase in bone mineral density in the non-weight bearing bones, the bones that were not exercised.

The older you are, the more benefits your bones have from exercise. Exercise of weight bearing bones builds mineral content, size, and strength.

Another important component of physical activity is that **exercise decreases diabetes and reduces the risk of non-insulin-dependent diabetes.** There are a number of studies showing the benefits of exercise on reducing the risk of diabetes.

With Diabetes you have a higher blood sugar level. Normally there is a decline in insulin sensitivity associated with aging, inactivity, and obesity. If you lose weight and increase your physical activity, you will increase your insulin sensitivity and decrease your risk of diabetes. Your pre diabetic condition may go away. **Diabetes is a chronic condition that greatly accelerates aging and often leads to premature death.**

There was a study done in Finland with 898 men. The men were subjected to moderately intense physical activity at high levels of cardio-respiratory fitness. It was found that after four years the more active individuals had a reduced risk of non-insulin-dependent diabetes mellitus of forty-four percent. That is very significant. That is **reducing your chance of diabetes almost in half just by increasing your physical activity.** If you lose weight, you do even better.

They also took the **overweight, high blood pressure people** in this group who had a family history of diabetes and who were engaged in moderate-to-intense physical activity at least forty minutes a week. **They reduced their risk of non-insulin dependent diabetes by fifty-four percent** compared to men who did not participate in such activities. What this is telling you is that **the fatter you are, the more out of shape you are, and the more risk you have, the greater you will benefit from exercise. It is never too late to start a physically active program.**

Talking about diabetes, in our teaching hospital we have an oncologist who slowly gained weight to the point where he developed hypertension and diabetes. What he decided to do surprised me, he went on an intermittent 5:2 fast, eating what he wanted for 5 days and 600 calories on his "fasting" days, and he lost 40 lbs. in 5 months. His hypertension went away and so did his diabetes. He was so impressed with the results that he did a grand rounds lecture for all physicians to know what can be done through intermittent fasting. He said it wasn't that hard, it's a goal like any other goal in life, you just don't eat, even if you are a little hungry on your fasting days.

An interesting thing that happens when you are physically active is you **increase your growth hormone level**. There was another study that measured the hormone levels, as well as the mineral levels and cardiovascular levels of endurance-trained postmenopausal women and sedentary women.

The endurance-trained postmenopausal women (probably greater than forty-five to fifty) had lower body fat, lower weight, and higher aerobic capacity. When normalized for weight, the bone mineral density was higher in the spine. The interesting part is the growth hormone level was increased.

Growth hormone is a hormone **associated with youth**. The theory is, the greater your growth hormone level, the more youthful characteristics you will have, such as greater lean body mass, less fat, more endurance, and a more youthful appearance. **Exercise naturally increases your growth hormone level.**

"Well, that's fine, but I've abused my body for all these years. This isn't going to do me any good." You are wrong!

The more you abused your body in the past, the greater your benefits. It has been proven over and over again in numerous studies that people in terrible shape can greatly benefit from physical activity. As a matter of fact, **they have the most to gain because they are the closest to the grave**.

Some of the **major impact studies** I consider important were done at Harvard University, Harvard Alumni Health Study, Cooper Clinic in Dallas, Texas, a very well-known aerobic and cardiovascular clinic, The Honolulu Heart Program, and the Finish twin study.

In the **Harvard study**, they took 17,321 men and studied them for approximately twenty-five years. They concluded that the **men who were vigorously active had about fifteen to twenty five percent less chance of dying**. Physical activity also decreased coronary artery disease, decreased high blood pressure, decreased non-insulin-dependent diabetes, decreased colon cancer, and increased life. One of the findings was that only vigorous activity had the remarkable difference in prolonging life. You had to expend about 1500 calories a week. Of the 17,321 men studied, there were 259 deaths of vigorously active individuals and 380 deaths from the non-vigorously active individuals. That's a big difference. There was a direct relationship between total physical activity and mortality. What does that mean?

That means, the more active they were to a certain limit, the less chance there was of them dying. One hundred twenty one more people died who were less active. That is almost one-third more deaths just because they were not engaged in physical activity.

At the **Cooper Clinic** in Dallas, Texas, they wanted to know if people who were initially in very poor condition could benefit from physical activity. They studied 9,777 men, ages twenty two to eighty, with a five-year follow-up. They found, as expected, people who were fit in the beginning and end had the lowest death rate. However, the **people who were unfit and became fit during the five-year follow-up study had a forty four**

percent reduction of the risk of death. This included all causes of death.

This should hit you between the eyes like a sledge hammer. **If you can decrease your chance of dying by forty-four percent, which is almost half, for all causes of death, wouldn't you jump on it?**

I would go out and buy a treadmill and start walking every day, or just get a good pair of sneakers and start walking in a safe neighborhood. How much more proof do you need to get off your butt and get going? Are you going to spend all your money when you get older on doctors, hospitals, and nursing homes? **It is your choice.**

Remember, exercise pumps out toxins. It prolongs life, and walking prolongs life. (Walking is even more fun if you go with a friend or family member and it's a great bonding time)

Let's get into the walking aspect. There was a study done in Honolulu of retired men by the Honolulu Heart Program. They took 707 non-smoking retired men from ages sixty-one to eighty one, and did a twelve-year follow-up. They recorded the distance these people walked. What they found is the more miles a person walked per day, the less was the chance of dying.

The men who walked less than one mile a day died two times faster than those that walked two miles a day. Their death rate was 40.5% versus 23.8% for the ones who walked two miles a day. What does that tell you?

Based upon this study and other studies I have reviewed and lectured on, **the magic number is two miles a day or more**. Guess what else they found?

The most common cause of death in the sixty-one to eighty one year old age group was cancer. The death rate for the people who walked less than one mile a day of cancer alone was 13.4%. For those who walked more than two miles a day, the death rate from cancer was 5.3%. That means **those who walked less than one mile a day had twice the chance of dying from cancer than those who walked two miles or more per day. What a difference just one mile makes**. Isn't that amazing?

That extra mile must trigger very important protective mechanisms in the body that keep your chemistry at balance, keep your body from going haywire, pumping out the toxins, increasing your cardiovascular fitness, increasing the oxygenation and nutrition to your cells.

Whenever I have a chance to learn from my patients about aging and longevity, I jump at the chance. Recently, I had a hair stylist who came in as a patient. I found out that she worked as a hair stylist in several adult living facilities, which I thought was quite a niche market for a beautician. I asked her about her observations of her older clients, questions primarily about their health, alertness, and what type of clients they made.

One interesting observation she told me was that **the hundred-year-olds** she does hair for, **are more active, walk better, and have a much better attitude about life than the seventy five to eighty year olds.** She also said **their minds and memories are better.**

Another thing that came out is that the hundred-year-olds were more resilient. They could overcome setbacks better and were much more pleasant to deal with than the sickly seventy five to eighty year olds.

She said that the younger ones who were sickly, less active, and not as alert mentally always worried about things. They talked about negative things all the time, worrying that they'd break their hip someday. Don't you know, they do break their hips. The ones who are sick always talk about being sick. The optimistic patients never seem to get as ill. The older patients seem to live for the moment. They enjoy life and they overcome obstacles through a positive mental attitude and an active lifestyle.

That is an interesting observation because it mirrors exactly what I have been finding in my research and my own observations. The more active you are, the less time you have to worry. The less you worry, the less chances you will have of developing a physical ailment that can greatly debilitate you and lead you to an earlier grave.

There is no reason to constantly worry about your physical state because you can do something about it.

There was another study done at the **Cooper Clinic** in Dallas, this one involving 25,000 men and 7,000 women. Researchers wanted to determine how people benefit from physical activity regardless of the shape they were in when they started. The study lasted nineteen years. Low, moderate, and high fitness levels were established for smokers, people with high cholesterol, high blood pressure, and other health conditions.

They found: 1. **That low fitness was an important precursor to mortality,** meaning the less fit you were, the greater your chance of getting ill; and 2. **That the protective effect of fitness held for smokers as well as nonsmokers, those with and without elevated cholesterol, and unhealthy and healthy persons.**

Everyone benefited from increased physical activity. People with low cardio-respiratory fitness benefited, as did moderate and high cardio-respiratory fitness, as determined by smokers and nonsmokers.

Every category improved with fitness. Those with normal blood pressure, moderately high blood pressure, and high blood pressure all systematically improved after an exercise program. The same thing was true for people who were generally ill all the time.

Remember my neighbor I mentioned at the beginning of this chapter, how I first met him when he was in his seventies? When I moved out of the neighborhood, he was well into his eighties and was in better shape than he'd been in his early seventies. The same observation I had on this one subject was observed at the Cooper Clinic with 32,000 subjects, which is the same observation my hair stylist patient noticed in her adult living facility centurions.

By the way, **did you know exercise also decreases breast cancer by twenty to thirty-three percent**? There are a couple of studies done about three years apart, one in Norway and another in the United States, which came up with these conclusions.

No matter what you say, some people will also be skeptical. You know why? Because they don't want to put in the effort. They think they are doomed. They think it is in their genes. They say, "Whatever happens, happens. I was destined to have cardiovascular disease . . . or cancer . . . or diabetes. . . ." They just give up.

I knew there would be objections to my findings, so I dug deep in the literature and found a **study done in Finland,** which was titled, **Relationship of Leisure Time, Physical Activity, and Mortality the Finnish Twin Cohort Study**. They knew that physical activity and fitness were believed to reduce premature mortality. What they did not know was **if genetic factors modified this effect**. (The, 'It's in your genes' hypothesis.) **They went on to study twins.** Twins are pretty much the same. They have the same parents, the same environment, and the same food. Identical twins have the exact same genes because they come from the same egg.

In this study done between 1977 and 1994, they took 7,925 healthy men and 7,977 healthy women from ages twenty-five to sixty-four. They classified them into conditioning exercisers and sedentary people. The conditioning exercisers walked vigorously for thirty minutes at least six times a month. The other group had no leisure physical activity. (I consider thirty minutes six times per month as mild exercise.) However, they considered that conditioning. Even with that minimal amount of effort, about one and-a-half days a week of vigorous walking thirty minutes, the results of the twins where one died during the studied period showed the odds ratio for death was sixty-six percent for occasional exercisers and forty-four percent for conditioning exercisers.

That means the people who walked vigorously at least thirty minutes at least six times a month had a twenty-one percent less chance of dying than the occasional exercisers; and, this was in twin pairs just walking thirty minutes six times a month.

When all the results from all the twins were compared, adjusted for age and sex, you had a seventy-one percent chance of dying as often as a sedentary exerciser if you were an occasional exerciser, and a fifty-seven percent chance of dying as often as a sedentary person if you were a conditioning exerciser. You had a twenty-nine percent less chance of dying if you exercised occasionally and forty-three percent less chance of dying if you exercised vigorously. To me, those are remarkable figures.

Based upon the twins studied, if you exercise vigorously only six times a month for thirty minutes by walking, you reduce your death rate chance by more than forty percent. The overall conclusion of this study was that familial factors did not explain the mortality differences by physical activity found in an individual-based analysis. **Occasional and conditioning twin exercisers had reduced risk of death compared to sedentary twins.**

I think you should re-read that last line several times until it sinks in. One interesting finding in this study when I reviewed the raw data was that **women seemed to do better than the men**. If you took the sedentary women and let's assume they had a 100% chance of dying at the end of the study, the conditioning women had a twenty-four percent chance of dying. That means they reduced their chance of death by seventy-six percent just by walking vigorously thirty or more minutes six times a month. It's amazing. Absolutely Amazing.

So wake up. **The only thing that is keeping you from increasing your life span is you.**

There have been other studies done that measure the benefits of lifestyle activity where they measured how active you were during the day. Today we use watches that measure if we did the recommended 10,000 steps in a day.

As expected, people who were more physically active during the day did better in their blood pressure, as well as in their body fat. What they are trying to show you is that it is not always necessary to have a structured physical activity program to get beneficial results from physical activity. However, the people in that group alone who did have a structured program had greater improvement in the cardio-respiratory fitness than those who were just more physically active in the daytime. On the world cruise my pulse rate on the treadmill, walking 3.5 mph for an hour each day, went from 98 to 87 beats per minute in a month. So, you will get more benefit out of a structured program that you do on a regular basis.

Movement is life.

If you don't move, you die.

It is as simple as that.

You get progressive decompensation if you don't move due to lack of muscle and joint stress, which eventually leads to rapid death.

These statements above are extremely important because they wrap up in a nutshell exactly what to you if you are not physically active. **If you do not have good muscle strength and coordination, you will trip**

and fall more and will not recover as easily. Several people on the world cruise tripped and fell on carpets, uneven sidewalks or ledges.

If your bones are weak because they have not been stressed, you break them more often, which will lead to further disability, bed rest, which can lead to pneumonia and eventual death, or you will have a greater chance of developing colon cancer, heart disease, and as shown in the Honolulu study, a fifty percent greater chance of developing all cancer just by not being physically active.

Did you know that **falls are the number one cause of injury in people 65 years old or older**? The risk of death 3 months after a hip fracture was 5 to 8 times higher? One in three adults age 65 and older falls each year and the cost to the US health system in 2010 for those falls was 30 Billion dollars. A walking program, as described in this book, could greatly reduce those falls and a dancing program even more.

On my world cruise, a number of people had to leave the ship because of falls. Those accidents ended their dream vacation. Some had broken bones, others infections, and others head injuries from their falls. One man that I know was admitted to a hospital in Singapore and later joined the ship in another country. They tripped on anything imaginable. I even saw one lady trip and fall down some carpeted stairs. We were afraid that she might have broken her ankle. At dinner the other night 2 out of the 6 people at the table had fallen during the cruise and one of them had a black and blue face, that's how the conversation came up when we asked him what happened.

During my Zumba class this morning, a medical emergency was called to the card room. People there sit and play bridge all day with no exercise. Two of the people that I know there are significantly overweight and walk real slowly. During my medical practice years, I've had 2 people die in front of me just sitting. They developed blood clots in their legs that went into their lungs. With the blood blow obstructed, oxygen couldn't get into the brain. We tried real hard to revive them, but they died. When you are inactive for a period of time, you need to balance that time with physical activity. Even pumping your feet up and down repeatedly while sitting, can make a big difference.

The World Health Organization (WHO) stated that "Levels of physical activity are decreasing and sedentary behaviors increasing with detrimental consequences" they mentioned cardiovascular disease, diabetes, hyperglycemia, hypertension and cancer along with obesity.

There has been some concern in the literature about over exercising, but in 2011 in the Journal of Sports Medicine a report about cyclists was published. The title was "Increased Average Longevity among the "Tour de France" Cyclists who did the grueling tour de France race between 1930 and 1964. Guess what they found? The age at which 50% of the general population died was 73.5 in that region of Europe vs 81.5 years for the "Tour de France" participants. **The extreme athletes lived 8 years longer.** I found similar data with Copenhagen joggers and Polish Olympic athletes. In the American Journal of Epidemiology June 2012 research article titled "Longevity in Male and Female Joggers:" The Copenhagen City Heart Study "Jogging was associated with significantly lower all-cause mortality". All-cause mortality means less death from all illnesses. Now that's a big deal.

Posture

I decided to include posture in this book because many people are not aware of the importance it has in our longevity program.

Why is posture important? It is important because it affects how our body ages and the health problems we may have because of poor posture. We need to be as erect as possible with our head straight, our shoulders back and our bellies tucked in.

Poor sitting and lying habits can affect our spine which can lead to deformities, degeneration and arthritis.

When you select a chair, sofa or recliner, make sure that the area you sit on from front to back is approximately the same length as the back of your knees to your back. You should sit with your back supported. The key thing is to maintain your core and preserve your spine. I had a doctor friend that purchased northern European furniture because it looked modern and “cool”. The problem was that the seat area was way too wide and he had to slouch a lot to lean against the back. He was trained in intensive care medicine. He had no idea that the sofa he was sitting on at home was ruining his spine while watching television or reading.

A new emerging exercise is Rucking. Rucking is where you exercise wearing a backpack filled with weights. It comes from the German work Rucksack, a backpack a lot of children in Europe wear to school. On my nightly walks, I used to see a man wear one of those heavy backpacks chugging along on his nightly walks. Based on my experience in rehabilitative medicine, why would someone want to add extra weight to their bodies? That extra weight has a deleterious effect on your knees, your spine and your posture because you have to lean forward to counteract the weight of the Rucksack.

When you are constantly slouched, the ligaments in the front of your spine become contracted. Contracted ligaments cause your spine to bow out in back like a humpback. This contraction leads to poor walking posture with your head leaning forward and down. The slouching can also permanently deform your spine, cause arthritis and decrease your lung cavity space so that you cannot breathe in as much air.

You need to oxygenate you tissues as much as possible when you are exercising. If there is less room for your lungs to expand, you cannot breathe in as much air. There is a lot of research done in this field but unfortunately most doctors, unless they are trained in rehab or pulmonary medicine, don't know anything about it. Too many pillows can also cause your neck and upper back to be deformed. Posture is important and we need to pay attention to it.

Pilates exercises and balance balls, are excellent for maintaining your core strength and balance. If you can strengthen your core, you will have less chance of falling and greater ability to recover from that fall. Pilates improves your posture, your balance and your stamina. It's best to do Pilates with a trained instructor to make sure you are doing them correctly.

There are different types of exercise as listed below: An exercise program that involves cardiovascular along with strengthening, is the best in my opinion. Because you progressively loose muscle mass as you age and especially after age 70, you need to build up that muscle mass constantly. You also need to increase your protein intake in order to build those muscles.

Your body absorbs less protein in the small intestine as you age. Younger people absorb 51% of consumed proteins while seniors only 45% or less. Therefore, seniors need to consume more protein to rebuild muscles. Ask your doctor if you have a medical condition. Studies have found that the lower your muscle mass, the greater is your chance of dying. A simple grip strength test done periodically will give you an indication of how you are doing in maintaining your strength. A grip strength test is also a good indicator of your overall strength. Interestingly, a very weak grip strength is also associated with dementia, according to a British study. Like the old saying goes, "Strength in mind, strength in body". Maybe those old timers were lot smarter than we think?

"Okay, okay. I've had enough data. Now tell me what to do." Here it is, but first ask your doctor.

1) Cardiovascular/Aerobic exercises such as running, bicycling, speed walking, elliptical machines, stair climbing, Zumba, step aerobics and others.

2) Strength building, core strengthening or bulking exercise like resistance training or weightlifting with free weights and gym machines; You can use heavier hand weights for large muscle groups and smaller ones for smaller groups. You can also use large resistance bands, which are essentially large rubber bands.

3) Load-bearing, such as walking, dancing, skiing, jumping or running. Load-bearing strengthens bones. Basically it's any exercise where you are standing on your feet.

4) Rowing, which involves compound movements; it is cardiovascular and muscle strengthening. If you use a rowing shell, you are exercising your legs, your upper body and abdomen all at the same time while enjoying

the water. Rowing machines in the gym, with a sliding chair, do the same thing without a water view.

5) Range of motion exercises such as Zumba, swimming, jumping jacks, Brazilian aerobics, Silver Sneakers Circuit or stretching. Swimming promotes range of motion throughout all your joints and it helps in resurfacing your joints as they become arthritic. It is one of the best exercises you can do but swimming does not strengthen load bearing bones.

Zumba is one of the best complex movement aerobic exercises that helps grow your brain along with dancing. Zumba involves movement of the arms, hands, legs, torso and feet all at the same time. It is different from step aerobics because you are also patterning your arms and hands. This movement is synchronized to music and a lot harder to do than it looks.

In Alzheimer's disease or Parkinson's, **complex movement training** is important for delaying symptoms or possibly stopping them. Complex movements use multiple pathways and provide redundancy. For babies, cross crawl patterning helps develop neuronal pathways. As the baby crawls from one place to another, he or she is growing their brain connectors. They use contralateral limb movement, such as right hand forward and left knee forward to train their neuronal pathways. In Zumba you also perform crass crawl patterns.

In Alzheimer's, Parkinson's or Lewi body disease, which is a form of Parkinson's, you want to have as much residual capacity to rely on as possible, in order to compensate for neuronal decay. You also want to increase your pulse and your brain circulation through aerobic activity.

Robert, a physician friend of mine, who was once the hospital chief of staff, started to develop Parkinson's disease in his early 80s. He immediately started a comprehensive exercise program, because he knew that exercise was effective in delaying Parkinson's.

People that go from simple forgetfulness, such as where did I put my keys or parked my car to noticeable Alzheimer's disease, have decreased brain circulation. Zumba gives you many of the same benefits as dancing. Aerobic activity, music therapy, balance, bone strengthening, ligament toning and coordination. You can watch Zumba on line or better yet attend Zumba classes. When you finish a half hour Zumba session you are sweating and feel good about yourself.

Dancing is one of my favorite exercises because it reduces stress and promotes joint movement, balance, endurance and brain growth. While you're dancing you are moving and having fun. You are building up new bone, strengthening your bones and reducing the risk of fractures. It can be a great social experience and you can do it well into your nineties.

Single retirees rarely get to touch someone. Touch is so important to our wellbeing that infants fail to thrive unless they are constantly touched. Through dancing you get to touch someone and connect briefly. That contact with another human being makes you feel better.

Since I am a ballroom, salsa and swing dancer, I have noticed a lot of healthy ladies and men in their eighties who are dancers. The good health of the older dancers lead me to write "**Dance to Live**". This book explains the health benefits one gets by dancing. By dancing you strengthen your bones, improve your balance, your memory, get cardiovascular exercise and increase your stamina. You also have a good time while interacting socially with others. The book is an easy read and the information will have you convinced that **dancing is one of the best forms of exercise you can have.**

I saw an article recently about a ninety-eight-year-old woman in Naples, Florida, who still dances several times a week. She had an interesting motto: "Smile awhile and while you smile, another smiles. Soon there are miles and miles of smiles. And life is worthwhile because you smile."

You should move as much as you can and reduce the stress on your joints by weight maintenance. Caloric restriction is one of the better ways to do it. Caloric restriction has significantly increased the life span of many species.

You should exercise your mind and body at the same time that you eat less. If you do that, you'll have a greater chance of living longer and know that you are living. If you stress your body through exercise, give it proper nutrients, and reduce your caloric intake, you'll have a better balance in the body's chemical reactions. Your body and mind will give you much better service.

Remember the studies I quoted with the rats who were mentally stimulated and the nuns who were mentally stimulated well into their nineties and had brains of young people, and the ninety year olds who increased their muscle strength by 174%. All of this is possible. And don't forget astronaut John Glenn who at 77 performed as well as forty-year-olds after his space flight.

Everything is possible if you get moving. What did **Jack La Lane,** the old guru of exercise, say? When he wrote his book at the age of eighty three, he said, "Old age is always twenty years away." He also stated, "There aint no fountain of youth. What you put into your body is exactly what you get out of it." How true that is.

And it is true in everything. What you put into your life, you get out. How you make your bed is exactly how you will sleep on it. What you sow is exactly what you will reap.

Now for the finale: **The Lenhart exercise program for longevity.** I came up with this formula after reviewing dozens of articles on physical activity for the lectures I give to physicians who took the anti-aging seminars. If you follow these examples, you will greatly, greatly increase your chance of living longer and healthier, as well as knowing that you are living by staying mentally alert and continuously stay excited about life. I see it in the 70, 80 and 90 year olds taking the world cruise.

1. Pump iron for 15-minutes to discomfort. That means, lifting various types of weights to stress your muscles. You can use free weights or the machines at the gym. For muscle building you increase the weight till you get discomfort. I generally have the weight set where I can only do 10-15 reps. Take rest breaks between muscle groups. For aerobic exercises with hand weights, you do more reps using less weight.

2. Change the muscle group each time you weight train. That means, change the muscles you are exercising. If you are doing upper body exercises one day, the next day do lower body exercises. It is not that difficult with machines and free weights to exercise most of the

muscle groups in the body. You can change the angles of fee weight for complex muscle groups.

3. Walk three miles in forty-five to sixty minutes, or to a slight sweat. Why is that important? You have to walk at a pace that actually stresses your body to a certain extent and gets your heart rate up. You have to sweat a little but not a lot. Just so you are slightly clammy. Sweating helps release toxins through the pores in your skin. It also builds up your cardiovascular fitness by increasing your heart rate and increasing your oxygenation. Remember to hydrate, hydrate, hydrate, eight glasses of water a day or half your body weight in ounces.

4. Use comfortable shock-absorbing walking shoes to reduce the ground reactive forces on your joints. One of the major problems people have with jogging or running is that they destroy their hips, knees or ankles. I strongly recommend walking with cushioned tennis shoes to reduce joint stress that can eventually lead to osteoarthritis. I do not feel it is necessary to run to exhaustion and destroy your joints at the same time. All that is really necessary is to walk at a good pace till you get clammy. In hot climates you're naturally going to sweat.

   It is also important to swing your arms while walking. Your left arm swings forward as you step on your right leg and your right arm swings forward as you step on your left leg. This cross crawl pattern is important for circulation and the nervous system.

5. Smile and think happy thoughts while you are exercising. It is very important to have a good mental attitude and positive mindset most of the time, based upon my observations and the observations of others, and of the people who live to be very old. The ones who

have the best mental attitude seem to do the best later in life.

6. Constantly stimulate your mind by learning. Your mental stimulation should also be varied, a diversity of things you learn stimulates different parts of your brain. Stress your mind by learning about a subject that you know nothing about. If you are into religion, social sciences, philosophy or politics also spend time learning about basic sciences such as astronomy, physics, biology, mechanics or technology. Crossword puzzles also work, but, make sure that they are on different subjects, like in trivia contests.

7. Do the above exercise combinations at least three times per week.

Hippocrates, the father of Medicine, stated **"Walking is man's best medicine".**

By the way, **to exercise in an airplane, stretch your legs out and pump your feet** up and down to increase your circulation and tone your muscles. If an airplane has something in front of your feet so that you can't stretch your legs out, ask to change your seat. I flew in an airplane from Europe once and the plane had an electronic box in front of my feet so I complained. The stewardess looked for an empty seat and changed my seat. If any aeronautical engineer is reading this book, do not design airplanes that limit passengers' ability to stretch out their legs in front of them.

Look at exercise as a job. It is **a job that you have to do whether you like it or not.** Work comes before pleasure.

Did you like getting up every morning to go to work? Did you like that boss that was always getting on your nerves? Did you like driving in heavy traffic each morning just to get to work? So, why did you work if you didn't like all those things?

You probably worked because you needed money to buy a house, buy a car, pay for a vacation, pay for your children's education, save for retirement and so on.

In retirement you need to use your body, just like that house, or else it will fall apart. If your body doesn't function properly, you will not be able to drive that car, take that vacation, enjoy your grandkids or go on those long RV trips or world cruises will you? You may not like getting up every morning to exercise, but, you didn't like getting up every morning to go to work either. Your job in retirement, if you chose to accept it, is to keep your body in good working order so that you can have fun and do things that you always wanted to do.

If you look at exercise as a job, you will just do it.

Don't let your body think that you're retired. If your body thinks your retired, it will kill you from the inside. In evolution there is little need of you past the reproductive and child bearing and raising years. It's more efficient to preserve younger people in order to propagate the species. That is why there is senescence where the cells stop dividing and get old, and apoptosis which is programmed cell deaths. If you trick your body by being active through exercise, it will think that you're still useful in evolutionary terms. Your body will help keep you young because it senses that you are still using it.

Exercise is work, but the rewards are well worth it.

You will not only add years to your life, but you will add quality of life to your years.

CHAPTER 5

Caloric Restriction

The data is clear. In experiments done on many species, less food, longer life. Caloric restriction is the only thing proven to extend life 30%.

When you observe people doing different things, such as walking, playing, moving from place to place, being involved in athletics, you'll notice a marked difference in activity and agility: The heavier they are and the more fat they have on them, the greater will be their ability to join the Polar Bear Club in Chicago. Just kidding. On a cruise ship, those people are always taking the elevator, even to go up one floor

What you actually see is less movement. **There appears to be a geometrical proportion in increased weight to decreased mobility and decreased agility**. How about coordination? How about shortness of breath with exertion?

What it boils down to be is the greater the increase in your fat level, the less you are able to move swiftly and efficiently. You may say that is obvious. Yes it is, but how many times have you thought about it, and how many times have you thought about the consequences this increased fat has on your entire life span?

On my world voyage we visited Kobe Japan. Kobe is a lovely city on the water with a beautiful waterfront and impressive Shinto temples. I remember riding my bicycle on the raised sidewalks and crosswalks. Kobe takes great care to protect its citizens from possible accidents while crossing a street. Kobe also takes great pride in its beef. Kobe beef is famous for being tender, flavorful and juicy. The reason that it tastes so good is because the beef is highly marbled with fat. The cows are not allowed to move and are constantly fed to build up their fat stores. The Kobe beef looks marbled because fat is in the muscles fibers. That marbling giving the beef its tenderness and flavor. It is also extremely expensive, some of the most expensive steak that you can buy anywhere in the world.

When you look at obese people, their muscles may also be micro marbled, just like Kobe beef. When the body injects excess calories, it converts the sugars from the calories into fat. Where does the fat go? It goes anywhere it can. First the energy from the calories is stored as glycogen, about 1600 calories, and then it is stored as fat. People with large bellies have large goblets of fat stored between their intestines. That area is called the omentum, where immune-regulation and tissue regeneration occurs. Fat can also go almost anywhere, your heart, skin, thighs, breasts, face, eye lids, neck and so on. People store fat in different locations based on their genetic predisposition.

Just like Kobe beef is the most expensive beef because the cattle are forced to not move in order to build up their fat stores. An obese person's fat also becomes incredibly expensive because of the hundreds of thousands they will have to spend just to stay alive later on in life. Excessive fat is responsible for the metabolic syndrome. Metabolic Syndrome is the new term for a combination of illnesses. High blood pressure, abdominal fat, high triglycerides, low HDL cholesterol and high fasting blood sugar. **Metabolic Syndrome is the number one disease in the western world followed by cancer.**

Cardiovascular disease, the number one killer, occurs as a result of metabolic syndrome.

If you are overweight, you have a significantly increased chance of developing a host of diseases from cardiovascular and diabetes to arthritis. You become a risk candidate if you need an operation because your chances of complications are much greater, as well as your chances of dying. Just think how hard it is to find a vein through all that fat? **If you take a hypothesis of movement is life, then less movement is less life.**

Do you want to live or do you want to live less? That is the question for you to decide.

Why do I have a chapter on caloric restriction? **Caloric restriction is so important in longevity that copping out of it, because it is difficult to do, would be a great disservice to you, the reader**. Original studies on caloric restriction were conducted in 1935 by Dr. Clive McCay, who was able to extend the life of rats 50% by severely restricting their caloric intake. Fifty percent. That's 50 percent. That's a lot.

I'm not talking about senile rats. I'm talking about active, vigorous, mentally alert rats. That research was largely ignored, although in the 1920s and '30s outstanding research was performed on various topics that are pertinent and directly correlative to our health problems today.

Let's get back to the general population and your observations. If you watch kids play on a playground, who does the most running, the fat kids or the skinny kids? Who moves around more from place to place? Who is more agile? Who gives the appearance of vitality and youthfulness?

If you could take the fat kid's movements and place them on top of an older person's movements, you would find that the obese children have activity levels of older, less mobile people, and middle-aged, overweight people have the same activity level of very old people. I think you're starting to get the idea that the fatter you are, the less physical life you have. Your mind may be willing, but your body won't move.

I saw a patient today who was thin, muscular, and lean. I asked him if his grandparents were also thin; he said yes, they were. I asked how long they lived; he said, "Oh, they lived to be a hundred." I asked about his parents; he said, "Well, they're well into their late seventies and they're still in perfect health." Then, he added, "But we eat an Indian-type diet of fish and chicken."

I had another patient come in and I noticed that he was also in very good shape, and this man was well into his sixties. I said, "You seem to be in phenomenal shape," I said. "How old was your father when he died."

"Did I say my father was dead?" he replied. "My father is ninety-one and he plays golf every day and goes dancing three times a week,"

"That's remarkable. Well, how old was your grandfather when he died?"

"Did I say my grandfather died?" he answered. "My grandfather is a hundred and twelve years old and just got married. Now he's expecting a child."

"That's really remarkable, somebody a hundred and twelve years old wanting to get married and start a family."

"Did I say he wanted to get married?"

The purpose of the above stories, one true and the other made up, is that if you are calorically restricted and are relatively thin, you will have a much more vigorous, active, and potent lifestyle into old age.

The other day, I was driving by the **Kids N' Kubs** baseball field in downtown St. Petersburg, Florida. I had some time after lunch, so I decided to stop by and watch these people play. They had a vigorous baseball game going on; good, solid hits to the outfield, line drives past the shortstop and second base and decent runs to first base. There were even spectators in the bleachers watching this exciting game.

I looked at every one of these players. **They were almost uniformly all thin.** A couple of them had slight potbellies, but nothing to be worried about. I talked to an elderly lady sitting next to the announcer and asked her about the team.

She said that "in order to qualify for the team, you have to be at least seventy-five years old, and those are the rookies". Her husband, who is the announcer, is eighty-eight. The president of the organization is ninety.

She pointed to a spry man walking fast after he picked up the bat from the batter. "He looks good and he runs good," she said. "He amazes me. And he's eighty-eight." I looked at the gentleman.

He was thin and lean. He had the body language of a thirty five year old. "A few have pot-bellies," the woman added. "They try to play, but they don't run as well."

Besides being active, the Kids N' Kubs are thin. They don't act "their age," they act young. Remember I stated movement is life, and the heavier you are, the less movement you are going to have and the sooner you'll fall into the grave.

What does the research show? I mentioned the original experiments from 1935, which were all but forgotten by modern medicine, then resurrected in the early seventies by **Dr. Roy Walford,** an M.D. researcher from California. You may remember him.

He was one of the participants, the medical person in the Biosphere II experiments near Tucson, Arizona. He had noticed that due to restrictions of the food they were trying to grow themselves **in the Biosphere, they were restricted to an 1800 calorie diet.**

He did repeated blood work on his fellow Biospherians and found that they were very healthy with the reduced caloric diet. They worked hard since they had to grow their own food to survive and they ate less. They lost weight and they felt good. The changes he saw in them were similar to changes he observed in other calorically restricted species.

The diet that **Clive M. McCay** developed in 1935 at Cornell University was low in calories but high in nutrients. This **high nutrient/low calorie diet** enabled his **rats,** which were fed a severely caloric-restricted diet to near starvation levels, to **live approximately 50% longer.**

Since the early seventies, Dr. Walford has been doing similar **experiments on mice**. In his mice experiments, a control group ate all they wanted and the caloric restricted group had **40% fewer calories** but all the nutrients they needed, including vitamins and minerals.

"What these mice have given mankind is perhaps the answer to a healthier, longer life," Dr. Walford stated "They live a remarkable one-third longer than their well-fed counterparts. This is the first and only intervention proven to extend maximum life span throughout the animal kingdom".

According to Dr. Walford, "It works all the way across the animal kingdom, calorically restricted one-cell organisms, worms, mice, rodents, rats, fish, all live a great deal longer, equivalent to let's say 150 to 160 years in humans. So, it would be very surprising if it worked all across the animal kingdom, then not in humans."

Dr. Walford also backed up his statements by the research he had done in Biosphere II, which was a sealed, three-acre dome with its own ecosystems. He noted that the humans in the Biosphere II dome showed the same extensive physiologic, biochemical, hormonal, and blood changes that rodents showed when they were calorically restricted.

In the **Biosphere II** experiment, Dr. Walford found that the **men showed an average weight loss of 26-pounds and the women 15-pounds by eating 1800 calories**. The **blood pressure of the individuals fell sharply. Total cholesterol also dropped 35%** on average. There was also noted a large drop in white blood cell counts, which indicated strong immune systems. (Similar findings were seen in people doing intermittent fasting.)

Calorie restriction has also more recently been found to activate Sirtuins, also known as SIRTs genes. These genes are involved in multiple biological processes, including DNA repair, cellular energy and slowing down the aging process. Exercise also activates SIRTs genes.

Some of the primary indications of youth are agility, coordination, and activity level. Dr. Walford tested those indicators in a log-rolling contest for mice. You must remember the concept two people balancing themselves on a log in water try to knock each other off. The one with the greatest balance, agility, and dexterity is the winner. Do you think an older individual would be as agile in a log-rolling contest as a younger individual? You would expect the coordination and reflexes of the older one to be much slower and his balancing ability to also be greatly diminished, wouldn't you?

The same thing held true for the mice. When the caloric restricted mice were pegged against the mice that ate all they wanted, the calorically restricted mice were thinner, had shinier coats, were more aggressive and agile, and were able to stay on a rolling log much, much longer than the fully fed mice.

In other words, although they were the same chronological age, their biological ages were markedly different. They acted as if they were young.

In humans, this makes a big difference whether you trip and recover on an uneven sidewalk, or you fall.

The mice that ate as much as they wanted were old and fell off the logs. Their reflexes were impaired. Their balance was impaired. Their coordination was impaired, and they lacked agility and endurance. The people that keep on falling on the world cruise have similar problems.

Now think about your experiences in observing other people. Think about people you have known who have been ill. Which show greater signs of youth, the overweight or the thin? How do they move? How are their reflexes? How quick are they? How fast do they walk?

The fewer calories you eat, the leaner you're going to be. As long as you eat a nutrient-rich diet, you're also **going to be healthy, agile, mobile, and experience greater physical performance** similar to that of your younger counterparts.

There was another experiment of interest done at the University of Wisconsin Primate Research Center, where I studied zoology, genetics and experimental psychology.

Dr. Rick Weindruch observed Rhesus monkeys that have been on a **caloric restricted (CR) diet**. The diet consisted of regular monkey chow not a scientific diet. Just like humans eat regular food, not scientifically crafted food, so, the monkeys ate regular monkey chow.

Since Rhesus monkeys live thirty to forty years, the experiment took a long time.

The study began in 1989 and findings in this 20-year longitudinal study were published in “Science” research journal in July 2009. The study stated that “In a population of rhesus macaques maintained at the Wisconsin National Primate Research Center, moderate CR (caloric restriction) lowered the incidence of aging-related deaths. At the time point reported, 50% of control fed animals survived compared with 80% survival of CR animals. Further, **CR delayed the onset of age-associated pathologies**. Specifically, CR reduced the incidence of diabetes, cancer, cardiovascular disease, and brain atrophy. **These data demonstrate that CR slows aging in a primate species**” Remember, monkeys are the closest relatives to humans since we are all primates.

After 20 years 50% of the control animals were still alive but in that same time frame **80% of the caloric restricted primates were alive. That is a huge difference.**

How would you like to improve your chances of having less diabetes, less cancer, less cardiovascular disease and less brain atrophy?

If you slow down aging, you have more time to enjoy life and do the things you want to. After all, don’t we want to be able to have as much fun as possible in our retirement? And remember what we did in the past?

Jessie, a thin, spry, attractive, happy, 94 year old lady that I interviewed in Twillingate, Newfoundland Canada **stated** "I do crossword puzzles all the time...it's good for the memory, **when your memory is gone, that's it, and you're gone**", how true. I saw a large print book of crossword puzzles next to her rocker. She said that she didn't eat much and got up out of her rocking chair to give me a copy of the exercises she did.

If you compare the pictures of a typical caloric restricted monkey and unrestricted monkey, who was able to eat what he wanted similar to a typical American diet, you will see a huge difference in appearance. A typical unrestricted monkey looked old, had a very thin fur coat with bald patches and a somewhat hunched back. The calorically restricted monkey had a youthful face, a lean body and a full thick fur coat. The difference in appearance between the caloric unrestricted and restricted monkey was startling. It was like looking at a 40 year old fit human, verses a 70 year old unfit sedentary balding human.

In the first edition of this book, the data was not all in and differences were starting to appear but after 20 years, what a marked difference in appearance, health and longevity in the calorically restricted primates. Just for curiosity, look at the pictures yourself on the internet. They were published in Science July 10, 2009. A picture is worth a thousand words.

I see this on the cruise ship, with people of the same age looking and acting markedly different.

By now I believe you're starting to understand how important caloric restriction is, as long as there are adequate nutrients. Vitamins, minerals, herbs, and essential nutrients will be covered in another section of this book.

The body only needs certain building blocks to function properly. Older individuals need more protein to maintain their muscles. When these requirements of trace minerals and vitamins are met, along with amino acids, and there is adequate bulk in our diet for motility of our gastrointestinal track (enough volume to push through our gut so we can have a normal bowel movement), the body will work efficiently.

We will be much healthier than the individual who eats excessively and clogs up his cells with pesticides, hormones, heavy metals, unnatural fatty acids such as trans fatty acids, micro plastics and thousands of other man-made chemicals that are hidden in our food chain.

Maintaining health is a perpetual ongoing process. It is a process at which we have to continuously work**. If you want to live healthy into your old age and not be "old" when you're old, you need to have a plan, and work that plan. Being "Young Old" is definitely better than being "Old Old". Your goal is to have your Biological Age be younger than your Chronological Age.**

Nature has certain basic laws that need to be followed. There are no quick fixes, no operations, and no magic pills. What effort you put into your anti-aging program, you will receive many fold over when you reach eighty, ninety, or one hundred and ten.

Dr. Walford was able to extend the life of his mice by a third by calorically restricting them to sixty percent of their normal caloric intake. The **standard American diet, SAD, consists of 2500 to 3500 calories, with some people eating considerably more than that.**

If we apply the same ratios of caloric restrictions to our diets, **we will be eating 1700 to 2000 calories per**

day. If we eat nutrient-rich, unprocessed, not chemically treated, pesticide-free foods, **we should be able to get the same benefits as all other animal species by restricting the diet. That is a longer, healthier life span by at least a third**.

A one third increase in our life span would allow us all to live between at least 100 to 120 years, some maybe even longer, up to 150. I definitely feel that young, healthy, active, mentally alert 100-year-olds are going to be plentiful in this century if they follow the longevity programs as described in this book.

In the Wisconsin Primate Research Center study, each caloric restricted animal's baseline food intake was reduced by 10 percent per month to reach a desired 30 percent reduction. This reduction would be about 1,750 to 2,450 calories per day for a typical person. It's a moderate reduction with proven health benefits in monkeys, our closest biological neighbors.

Remember, you reap what you sow. If you sow healthy seeds in a lean, chemically pure, fit body, you will reap a long, healthy, active, alert, joyful, fun life into a very young old age. **There are the old-old and the young-old. You want to be in the young old category.**

So where do you start? **A good place to start is to eat small meals throughout the day and not eat anything after a supper.** Another thing you could do is eat a **big meal at lunchtime and a light meal or snack in the early evening**, preferably consisting of either fruit or a light salad with a little extra virgin olive oil or canola oil and apple cider vinegar.

You could also have some protein consisting of beans, broiled cod or salmon, or free-range chickens (those whose feed has not had hormones or arsenic added). The important thing to remember is to eat early, as close to 5 as possible, and keep your evening meal very light. It's best to eat your main meal during lunch if possible. **Just not eating after supper is a good start toward caloric restrictions**. My patients that did not eat after 5 PM lost weight.

If you eat twice a day, have a large breakfast and a late, say 2-3 PM, lunch, which I call "Lupper". Talk to your physician if this is appropriate for your health condition.

We will go into nutrient recommendations further on into this book. You will have to figure out for yourself how to greatly reduce your caloric intake by eliminating high fructose corn syrup adulterated foods and drinks, deep-fried foods, pastries and sweets and substituting nutrient-laden foods consisting of primarily pesticide-free fruits, vegetables and nuts.

Yes, you can occasionally splurge and treat yourself as long as you **maintain a regular caloric-restricted diet of between 1750 to 2450 calories. Occasional palate alteration is not going to hurt you that much.**

So plan ahead to a happy, active, joyful, alert retirement with a superb quality of life.

Don't depend on that magic pill, or rely on having your blood transfused with young blood or plasma as a last ditch effort to stay young.

Depend upon yourself now while you can. Stop eating junk. Reduce your calories drastically and you will reap the benefits at the later stages of your life, where it counts the most.

You, too, can be like the 91 year old piano player on the world cruise, stealing the piano away from me at 7 AM in order to practice. You can also be like the eighty-eight year old Kids and Cubs baseball player who acts and behaves like he's thirty-five, full of energy and vitality, enjoying his life to the fullest.

Chapter 6

Happy Things to do in Healthy Aging

This chapter did not exist in the "Seven Secrets of Anti-Aging" book. When talking to retirees, I noticed that some did not have hobbies or interests outside of their work. Many professionals were so engrossed in their work that they had little time to develop other interests. By reading this chapter, you may get some ideas of things to try that will bring you pleasure in retirement and a happier life.

As previously noted, Studies have shown that one of the most important components of longevity is social interaction. Humans are social creatures and social interaction with others has a lot to do with how well we age. People that are socially engaged through activities and that have social networks seem to have a happier and healthier retirement. We need to be with other people.

We **humans are creatures of emotion**. We make major decisions based on emotion. Our religious beliefs, the partner we marry, our political affiliation and our career and leisure time activities all have an emotional component. When we retire we want to have as many positive emotions as possible and reduce or eliminate negative emotions. We start to focus on "living happily". We accentuate the positives and try to eliminate the negatives in our lives.

What does "to live" mean? For me it means passion. That spark and life that stimulates us to go on and achieve new goals, new pleasures and joys. Something to look forward to. It means to spark new desires yet to be fulfilled. It is an intense burning to achieve something or do something that you find infinitely rewarding. And note, there's a big difference between "existing" and truly "living".

To "live" means reaching beyond the ordinary, beyond just mere existence. It means exploring those passions that before retirement you never had the time to do because ordinary life got in the way. Now is the time to let go, explore and enjoy those things you dreamed of doing. This is the final quarter of the life game, have fun and enjoy the "Happy things to do in Healthy Aging".

Remember that all sedentary activities have to be balanced with active activities to keep your body moving. On the world cruise I see Bridge Players sitting all day on their butts playing bridge. That's all right as long as they add an hour or more of exercise to their routine.

1. **The Morning Walk** – Taking a walk the first thing in the morning is a good thing to do. It gets you moving, smell the fresh air, watch the sunrise, burn calories and makes you feel good about yourself.
2. **The Night Walk** – Everyone loves a sunset. Why not combine watching a sunset with a half hour walk before and after the sunset? The colors become spectacular after the sunset.
3. **Going to the Gym** – A friend of mine goes to the Y several times per week and loves the classes. A morning aerobics or Zumba class is a good way to get moving and get some cardio and range of motion exercises in. In Canada they have huge gym complexes with everything imaginable in them. Winters are long and cold in

portions of Canada so they build huge gym complexes in order for people to stay healthy. In my building there are always people working out on the treadmill, weight machines or free weights. They enjoy staying in shape, and keeping their muscles toned.

4. **Bike ride** – We have many bicycling clubs in St Petersburg Florida. I belong to a rollerblade and biking group and we have different rides three times per week. We meet up at various locations and do 11-15 mile rides. I also used to ride my road bike with serious gearheads. You do not have to go fast, just get out and enjoy bike riding at whatever level you feel comfortable. It helps if your city has numerous biking trails like they have in Sopot Poland, Berlin, Singapore or Netherlands.
5. **Scripture Study Group** – Many people get involved in scripture study. They want to understand their religion better. The inner peace that people find from religious studies makes them happy. Spirituality and having a connection with God is very important to them. In many parts of Asia the writings of great spiritual leaders are incorporated into everyday life. People strive to encompass those philosophies for a more harmonious peaceful life.
6. **Sailing** – Being anywhere by the water makes a lot of people happy. Many of my friends love to go sailing on beautiful sunny windy days just like I do. Albert Einstein was a big fan of sailing, that's where he did his most inspirational thinking. Walter Cronkite was also an avid sailor and so is Morgan Freeman. Yacht racing can be challenging and a lot of fun too.
7. **Bridge club** – In Florida there are many Bridge card clubs at the Masters level. People find Bridge to be an enjoyable strategic card game that can be socially engaging as well. A word of caution about Bridge. Bridge can be addictive and people sometimes play 8 hours at a time. There are numerous books written on Bridge strategy, how to bid and play duplicate bridge. The

better your memory, the more competitive you can become in bridge. From talking to bridge club leaders, the clubs sort of peter out when people are in their early 80s. On my world cruise you see the same people sitting all day playing bridge. They do not do anything else except maybe take an excursion on a bus. All this sitting around is not good for your circulation or your health. You need to balance the mental work playing bridge with physical activity. Your body is not designed to sit all day, especially at an older age. The reasons are explained in my physical activity chapter. Mahjong is gaining in popularity. Bridge is fading slowly since younger people no longer play it because of computer and internet games.

8. **Kayaking** – Kayaking is something that I like to do on a regular basis. It is one of the cheapest forms of boating that you can do. Kayaks are portable and can be enjoyed on lakes, rivers and oceans. Join a kayaking club and have fun being on the water. If you live in a condo, there are foldable, light polypropylene kayaks that fit under a bed
9. **Tennis / Pickleball** – Tennis is very popular in warm climates. It is an aerobic and social activity requiring strategy and skill. Make sure that you are playing on soft courts not concrete. Your knees will last much longer if you play on har-tru green clay courts. In St Petersburg Florida we have pick up round robin tennis Monday, Wednesday, Friday mornings where you switch doubles partners every 3d game. It's a no brainer, get out of bed, be there by 8:30 and there is a group of tennis players waiting to play. **Pickleball** is a transition from tennis into a smaller court and is played a lot in retirement communities along with Ping Pong. Pickleball has exploded in popularity; it hones your reflexes and response time, allows you to be outside, socially engaged and appears to be less stressful on the knees than tennis.

The learning curve for pickleball is shorter than tennis and it's a good way to be active and make new friends.

10. **Baseball league** – All cities have baseball leagues. Find a senior league and start playing. Senior slow pitch softball may be a good option.
11. **Golfing group** – Retirement and golfing go hand in hand. You will find hundreds of communities designed around golf courses in Florida, Arizona, New Mexico and other retirement areas. They will also have aerobics classes, a gym, guest lectures and excellent dining facilities.
12. **Walking / Hiking** - In Europe and in mountainous areas throughout the world, there are clubs that go out on weekends hiking. Those people love being outdoors in nature and hiking the hills and mountains near them gives them a sense of being part of nature. Entire vacations can be spent traveling to hiking destinations throughout the world such as the Milford Trek in southern New Zealand, the Rocky Mountains in the USA or in the Andes of South America. My niece in Europe loves to go hiking in the mountains. She belongs to a hiking group and every weekend there is a trip planned somewhere for all day hikes. Hiking is a great way to exercise and experience nature as you watch the spring flowers bloom or fawns frolic in the meadows. On one of my RV trips to Shenandoah National Park, one of my campsite neighbors just came back from trekking the trails in northern Vietnam. He told me that he had hiked some of the best trails in the world. When I asked him which he liked best, he said that Canada has some of the best hiking trails. He liked Banff National Park and the Rocky Mountains both in Canada and the USA. Walking in city or county parks is something you can do several times per week with a friend or alone. The move it or lose it chapter explains why 2 or more miles each time is optimum for longevity.

13. **Dancing** – My book "**Dance to Live**" points out all of the health benefits of dancing. In my opinion dancing is one of the best activities for aerobic exercise, balance, coordination, mental enhancement, stress reduction and social engagement all wrapped up into one fun filled activity. In my area there are large weekly east coast swing dances with lessons, Argentine tango, Carolina shag, salsa, square and contra dances and multiple ballroom dances at various studios. Dancing involves multiple complex neuronal pathway therefore enhancing your memory reserve. The more reserve you have, the greater your chance of delaying Alzheimers disease. I know a couple in their late 70's that dances 5 nights a week. He picks her up and twirls her around as if they were 20 again. I also dance with a lovely 87 year old lady who is convinced that dancing keeps her young, and I agree.
14. **Date Night** – Just as dating was important as you were raising children, dating is important in retirement. It keeps you engaged with your partner having fun doing activities you both enjoy together. Your date could be the traditional dinner and a movie or, an evening performance at the theatre or symphony. Anyplace where both of you have times to connect and enjoy each other will work just fine.
15. **Girl's night out** – Girls need their night out, just to be girls again and have fun without worrying what the guys think. Friends of mine get together weekly leaving they guys behind. Many don't have partners anymore and going out with other ladies allows them to look good and have fun. They also get to catch up on the latest news about their friends, and maybe help each other with problems that arise.
16. **Hanging out with other guys** – Guys love to get together in their man caves and solve the world problems. They also love to get together to talk about their hobbies and sport teams. On my world cruise a

group of older guys would sit together at a large table at breakfast and chat mostly about all the RV trips they took. Male bonding over a common interest.

17. **Fishing** – I've known many a fisherman that gets up at 4AM to catch that incoming tide or go out on their flats boat. Fly fishing can become a passion for some people and they will travel half way around the world to do it. Off shore fishing is very popular in Florida just like lake fishing.
18. **Shooting and Archery** – From clay pigeon shooting to target practice, shooting has been a hobby and sport for thousands of years. Archery, the original form of shooting, is still popular.
19. **Jewelry making** – A retired Psychiatrist I knew had an entire room dedicated to bead jewelry making. She loved to make glass and colored stone necklaces and bracelets. She found it to be relaxing as well as creative.
20. **Painting, pottery and ceramics** – Many people have always wanted to paint but never had the time to do it. Now is the time to take that art class and learn what you can do. Making stained glass windows is another hobby that retirees are taking up along with throwing clay pots and decorative ceramic glazing. If you take a long cruise, there are water coloring, sketching and knitting classes offered on the sea days. A good friend of mine took a sketching class offered on the sea days on the world cruise. By the end of the cruise I couldn't believe how good the drawings of humans in various positions were.
21. **Knitting and Sewing** – A friend of mine developed a second career after retiring designing specialty yarns and writing knitting books that became very successful. Look for a sewing meet up group and explore designing your own clothes.
22. **Racquet Ball** – Just like tennis, racquet ball is a competitive aerobic sport that gives you fast paced

work out and an opportunity to socialize. **Badminton** can also be very competitive.

23. **Book Club** – Reading is very popular for many people. In St Petersburg, Florida we have the "Festival of Reading" that brings authors from everywhere to talk about their books and what inspired them. Books clubs get together to select a book of the month to read and discuss that book at their next meeting. The meetings are generally in someone's home and enjoyable.

24. **Travel Club** – In retirement most people love to travel. They want to visit places that they have read about to experience them personally. Travel Club members exchange stories and provide good information as to where to go, what to avoid and what to do at travel destinations.

25. **Adventure Travel** – Adventure travel takes travel to another level. It can be anywhere, from exploring Patagonia on long wilderness hikes, to seeing an Orangutan preserve in Thailand. You can be riding your bicycle for 50 mile/80 km per day touring Ireland, hiking up a mountain, or paddling down some river in New Zeeland. On my transatlantic cruise, I met an Australian couple on their way to hike the Camino de Santiago from France through northern Spain. They had traveled all over the world. If they like a place, they will stay there for weeks. A former nurse and her husband love to go on Safaris in South Africa. Another couple chases sun and lunar eclipses everywhere. Go on line and search Adventure travel, you may be surprised.

26. **Gardening** – There is nothing like feeling dirt between your fingers as you plant that seedling. It makes you feel like part of nature making something grow. You watch that seed pop out of ground and become a beautiful flower. Some people love Bromeliads, others orchids or roses. Growing Bonsai trees can be a real challenge. Join a gardening club. If

you grow your own vegetables, you will have pure food for your body to enjoy.

27. **Cooking Club** – My best friend loves to cook and bake. She finds cooking a variety of good tasting dishes rewarding and a diversion from her day job. When she bakes, she gives it all away not to gain weight. The creative process of blending spices and ingredients allows her to relax. Off course we tell her how wonderful her cooking is. Cooking Clubs explore a variety of dishes and styles. They re-define subtleties in flavors that most of us never experienced. You can also go to a Culinary School.

28. **Volunteer Organizations** – If you want another purpose in life, give back to society. Help those in need get back on their feet. Being a volunteer for worthy causes can be very rewarding and a good use of your spare time. Philanthropy, if you have the resources, can be an engaging and rewarding endeavor.

29. **Docent** – Some people just love museums. Being a docent and knowing everything about the artist can be a fulfilling volunteer activity. Historical locations and buildings also have docents. During my world voyage I sat with a gentleman who is a docent in the historical section of Annapolis Maryland. I asked him what got him interested in becoming a docent. He told me that he was a chemical engineer and had lived in Singapore on assignment. While in Singapore he became interested in its history and its development from a fishing village into a world class city. He said that he always had an interest in history. When he retired, he thought that it would be nice to share his passion with others. He found Annapolis history fascinating and thought his interests and knowledge would be appreciated by others. He studied interesting events, read old archived newspapers and brought that history to life as he guides tourists through famous residences. In St Petersburg Florida we have docents at the Salvador

Dali Museum, they share their passion about the artist with museum visitors.

30. **Dog walking** – People that love dogs, Love dogs. Did I say Love dogs? Help a pet sitter on a part time basis so that she can take a vacation and fill in when she is too busy. You can also get involved in dog rescue or raise puppies for guide dog organizations.

31. **Senior Learning College** – This is a big one. **Lifelong Learning is very important** for continued brain development. In St Petersburg, Florida we have ASPEC, Academy of Senior Professionals at Eckerd College and OLLI, Osher Lifelong Learning Institute. USF University of South Florida has free noncredit college courses and St Petersburg College has lifelong learning classes. Every community has lifelong learning. My 83 year old sister in Poland learned how to operate a computer at such a class and has become a virtual traveler and student.

32. **Continued Education** – If you are a professional, it's good to keep learning in your field. Personally, I go to as many continuing medical education lectures that I can. My routine involves going to 1- 2 hours of continuing medical education (Grand Rounds) each week. The lectures keep me informed of the newest developments in medicine. The lectures are also a good way to interact with people that have similar education. The post seminar lunch conversations can become intellectually stimulating and lots of fun. Like my sister, a former math teacher, said "I exercise my brain".

33. **Mentoring program** – Many new business entrepreneurs and professionals need mentoring to become successful. They could use your expertise to become better in their profession. You will feel better because you have helped someone achieve their dreams. Big Brother, Big Sister and the Scouts are good organizations to help young people flourish.

34. **Volunteering in animal shelters** – Help an abandoned or stray animal find a good home. Dog rescue programs, Friends of Strays and the Humane Society always need volunteers.

35. **Hospital Volunteer** – Hospitals need volunteers of all kinds. You can be running the gift shop or assisting nurses and patients. Being a Hospice volunteer can be very rewarding. Get involved and find out what volunteers your local hospital needs.

36. **Church Organizations and Civic Clubs** – Churches need volunteers to help the church community flourish. You can get involved in anything from education, church fairs, after school care to meals on wheels for the elderly and sick. Civic Clubs get you involved in the community and help others.

37. **Special Interest Meetup groups** – Go online and type in meetup groups in your area. You will be surprised as to the large variety of groups. At the Villages near Ocala Florida, there are over 3,500 resident run clubs. It's a good way to become socially engaged with others.

38. **Writers group** – If you have always wanted to write a book, find a writers group and learn how the process works. You will benefit from the knowledge of other authors.

39. **Inventors Club** – We have one in Tampa Bay. Members discuss their ideas, show prototypes, get feedback and learn how to patent and protect their inventions.

40. **Car restoration** – For car buffs, restoring and old car is fascinating. You can see this rust bucket become a beautiful piece of art that you can show off at car shows. The same holds true for old boat or motorcycle restoration. I've met Brits restoring old trains.

41. **Fashion Club** – An old friend of mine loved to watch fashion and designer shows on television. Get together with likeminded people and follow the latest fashion trends or create your own gowns.

42. **Antiquing** – Making the old, new again. People love antiques. There is a television show just dedicated to that. There are flea markets and antique fairs all over the place. Someone that I knew spent a lifetime collecting things of value and now he is selling his valuables on line to other collectors. A lady I know finds old furniture and makes it look new.

43. **Investor groups** – Investor group meetups are in most retirement areas. Be careful and use hypothetical purchases for a long time before you start throwing real money into the game. The group meetups are good for learning and discussing investment options.

44. **Symphony** – If you love classical music, going to the weekly symphony or pops concerts is an enjoyable way to spend Saturday afternoon or evening. Opera and Ballet are other options.

45. **Theatre** – Community Theatre exists everywhere. Become an actress, actor, stage hand or just support the theatre company by going to their plays. I love going to see live theatre, either on Broadway or at a local playhouse.

46. **Playing your instrument in a band** – Many of you were in a high school band. Did you know that there are marching bands for former band members? In St Petersburg, Florida we have "The Second Time Arounders" Marching Band. If you played an instrument or were a majorette in high school, find a group of people and jam with them. In Stephenville Newfoundland I heard "The folks on the bay", a group of fiddlers, guitar players, banjo players and drummers that played a variety of folk and Irish music.

47. **Learning a musical instrument** – Learning to play a new musical instrument can be very

challenging and rewarding. The dedication and time required can make your brain grow younger. Mastering a musical instrument is as much of an anti-aging activity as dancing or walking. Recent data shows that playing a musical instrument may delay the onset of Alzheimer's disease or make its progression slower. The extra neuronal pathways that are created through playing a musical instrument seem to have a protective effect on the brain.

48. **Choir or Choral group** – My mother loved to sing in the church choir. In my area we also have the "Madrigals", a choral group that sings old English Capella songs in the Madrigal style. If you love to sing, join your church choir or a choral group.

49. **Wine tasting** – Wine tastings are available in wine stores and at private clubs and restaurants. If you enjoy fine wine, like my uncle did, go and find your perfect dinner wine and wine for special occasions. It's a good way to socialize and meet new people to do other things with. Just don't over indulge and stay within the legal limits.

50. **Shuffle Board Club** – St Petersburg Florida was once world famous for its shuffle board courts. Guess what? Shuffle board is coming back, the old shuffle board courts are filled with retirees in the daytime and young people on dates Friday and Saturday night.

51. **Sailing Race Official** – This is a niche hobby that few people ever thought about. Yacht racing requires people to organize and run the regattas. If you love being on the water, have you ever thought about running sailboat regattas or powerboat predicted log races?

52. **Flying Club** – In Lakeland Florida and Oshkosh Wisconsin the EAA, Experimental Aircraft Association, has yearly fly-ins. People from all over the world go there to see the latest developments in ultralights, sport planes, gliders and personal aircraft.

The daily air shows are spectacular. Last year I saw a jet powered biplane do amazing aerial acrobatics. Local airports all have flying clubs you can get involved in.

53. **RV travel – Recreational Vehicles** and retirement go together like peanut butter and jelly. A great portion of this book was written in my RV traveling in Northeastern Canada and Western United States. I met fellow RVers that told me of other places that I may want to visit. One couple that I met had been full time RVers for 10 years and saw every part of the US, Alaska and Canada twice. They told me that they liked the National Parks and wildlife sanctuaries the best. In mid-January at the Florida Fairgrounds in Tampa, we have the Florida RV Supershow, one of the largest in the world. In the fall, in Dusseldorf Germany there is a huge RV show, The Caravan Salon.

On a transatlantic cruise I met an American couple who for the past 15 years, had lived all over western and eastern Europe in an RV. They come back to the states on a cruise ship every couple of years in the fall, rent an apartment and a car in Sarasota Florida for 6 months and then take another cruise ship back to Europe in the spring. There are many RV travel clubs you can join, as well as caravans that do all the planning for you. Go on line and read the blogs of people traveling in RV's. On my world cruise, many passengers have an RV or used to have an RV. A number of couples that I met travel in their RV in the summer and on cruise ships in the winter. Others migrate from the northern cold winter states and Canada to Florida or Arizona. In Europe and England you see a migration to southern Spain in the winter where it's warmer.

54. **Boating Cruising Club** – Boat owners like to get together at various yacht clubs and marinas, socialize and have dinner. It's a good way to meet other boaters and see the area. You can go cruise either in a

power boat or a sailboat. Some cruising clubs are just for Sailboats and others have both sail and power. There are also on line meetup boat clubs. People with similar live aboard trailer boats, such as Rosborough, Cape Dory or Ranger pocket cruisers, have on line meet up groups and get together in various cruising locations.

55. **Ship Cruising** – The cruise industry just keeps on growing with cruises being offered all over the world. Many people like cruising because you get to see different parts of the world in a floating hotel. Just remember to walk the decks or go to the fitness classes on board to maintain your weight and stay in shape. The relocation cruises have a very high percentage of retirees on them from all over the world. What I find interesting is talking to all those fascinating people, what they did in their careers, and their current interests in retirement. If you sit with random people at large tables, you will learn a lot about peoples interests, which in turn may spur on your interests.

This morning I sat with Jan, a 70 year old molecular biophysicist who dove 2,000 feet under the ocean in a research submarine studying tube worms living by volcanic vents. She spends over 180 days a year cruising in ships which includes around the world cruises. If you like quiet cruising, consider going on a cargo ship with passenger cabins. Some people even live full time on cruise ships. Food, entertainment, room service, and social interaction – sounds like a winning combination to me. On my world cruise, I've met quite a few people that do 4-6 month world cruises year after year. A man in my aerobics class has done 14 of them. When he retired from Silicon Valley, he moved to Florida so that he could just rent a car and drive to the cruise terminal in Ft Lauderdale.

A married couple, in their early 60s, retired in their 50s, just to be able to RV and travel on cruise ships while they still had energy to explore. They were both engineers, had no kids, saved their money, invested wisely and planned for their retirement all along. Yes, it's possible to retire early if you plan for it. If you book your cruise 6-12 months ahead of time, then you have something to look forward to. You will be anticipating something different in your life, something interesting and rewarding.

56. **Aerobics Classes** – Fitness clubs and the YMCA offer these popular classes regularly. From the morning stretch to Zumba to body pump aerobics, it's a good way to stay in shape and be motivated by your fellow participants. On my world cruise, I go to Zumba classes regularly because they makes me move and sweat. The best part is you sweat to the rhythms of music, moving your arms and legs at the same time to a constant beat.

57. **Swimming** – Swimming is one of the best exercises you can have. Most retirement communities have pools. A daily swim can make you feel refreshed and all limbered up. You could join a local swimming club.

58. **Learning another language** – You have always wanted to learn German, Italian, French, Chinese or Spanish haven't you? If you really want your brain to grow, learn another language in retirement.

59. **Cultural Immersion in another society** – What better way is there to learn about another society than actually living there for a few months? You experience their food, entertainment, culture and how they think. It's a good way to develop an appreciation for other cultures and a different perspective. I knew a lady that would rent out her Anna Maria Island Florida condo and rent an apartment in Paris. The rent she got for her condo on Anna Maria Island payed for her Paris rental and living expenses.

60. Woodworking – Furniture Building

Having a small woodworking workshop in your home can be very relaxing and creative. There are woodworking clubs that have machines that you can use for your creative furniture, rocking chair or baby crib projects.

On my world cruise, I met a retired nuclear submarine captain that spends 6 hours a day in his wood shop. When I asked him what he built, he showed me photographs of showroom quality furniture. The inlaid wood, the type of wood chosen, the attention to detail were exquisite. Who would have thought that such quality furniture could be manufactured in someone's garage?

61. Model Plane Flying and Car Racing – If you can't get the big plane, get the small plane and fly it at a local model plane club. One of my neighbors had two model jet planes in his garage that flew 400 miles (643 kilometers) per hour. While bicycling in Singapore, I saw a race track with many turns just for model cars. There were people working on their cars in the covered area just like you see on full size race cars. Singapore has miles of contiguous parks on the Ocean labeled A through H. The tree filled parks, made from reclaimed land, have a beautiful garden area with domed eco systems, excellent wide shaded bike trails, a wake boarding lake, a kayak and dragon boat racing lake, baseball, golf and numerous boating clubs including a huge youth sailing IOD dingy club. It's a spectacular playground for its citizens.

62. Model Sailboat Racing Club – Radio Controlled sailboat racing is just as competitive as racing big sailboats. The boat class size is standardized and the wind is the same for everyone.

63. Dining out – If you like to sample different restaurants, dining out is a good way to spend time with your spouse or friends. Some people just love the subtleties of foods and wines. You could join an epicurean club along with a wine club to develop your taste buds. Small portions along with exercise are essential if you love food.

64. **Bowling league** – Bowling is a good way to get involved in a group activity or just have fun with your loved ones and friends. There are bowling leagues everywhere.

65. **Sporting events** – Many retirees like going to sporting events. Baseball, Hockey, Football, Soccer and Basketball are popular spectator venues. The afternoon baseball games are filled with retirees having a great time. Hot dogs and cracker jacks are just as popular now as they were 75 years ago.

66. **Skiing** – One of my friends is over 80 years old and skis like a teenager. Tampa Bay has one of the largest ski clubs in the country. Many northerners retire here and they like to ski. There are trips all over the world.

67. **Parachuting** – Some people like the thrill of jumping out of a perfectly good airplane at least once in their lifetime. I was surprised on a recent transatlantic cruise by how many people raised their hands when the comedian asked them if they ever went parachuting. On my world cruise over 20 people signed up to parachute in Hawaii. I have something against jumping out of a perfectly good airplane, so I did not participate. In Cape Town, South Africa another group went paragliding off the top of Lionhead Mountain.

68. **Experimental Aircraft building** – A friend of mine build an ultralight airplane in his garage that he fitted with pontoons to use on a lake in central Florida. The EAA (The experimental aircraft association) has a large variety of planes at their shows. Another friend goes to the EAA shows in Lakeland Florida in the winter and to Oshkosh Wisconsin in the summer. These shows

feature anything from the latest in electronics to jets, sailplanes, ultra-lights, light sport planes and gyrocopters.

69. **Homemade racing boats** - Friends of mine built small 8 foot race boats that competed with highly tuned 10 horsepower engines on local lakes. There is a large variety of classes of small boats you can race, just like there is in car racing. On my cruise to Japan, I saw a giant stadium in an inlet used for "Kyotei", which is small boat racing. The stadium was as large as ones used for car racing, except that it was located on water. Kyotei is one of Japan's four public sports.

70. **Car racing** – If you love speed, watching car racing can be an exciting sport to follow. In St Petersburg, Florida we have the St Pete Grand Prix. It is an open wheel Indy car race similar to the Formula 1. People from all over the world come to watch this event and it is televised globally.

71. **Model building** – Model building is an art form that requires a great deal of attention to detail. You may enjoy the process of starting with nothing and creating this beautiful scale model sailing ship or plane. Model building just like jewelry making is relaxing to a lot of people.

72. **Bird Watching** - is probably one thing you never thought of. There is a whole group of people (birders) that communicate with each other constantly on the internet about rare species of birds that they have seen. They will drive hundreds of miles to find a rare bird that someone has spotted. I have run into them many times at nature preserves carrying large cameras with monopods so they can take just the right photo of that exotic bird. They will post that photo on the internet for other birders. Some people also like to record bird songs with high quality portable audio recorders. Before my last cruise, I recorded bird songs that I hear every

morning where I live. Listening to their recorded singing voices makes my cruise ship cabin feel more like home.

At breakfast on my recent transatlantic cruise, a 79 year old man from Sun City center Florida told me that he and his wife have been birders for a long time. They told me of going birding to South Africa, spending a month in Tasmania, the Texas birding festival, the Rio Grande valley and of bird migratory patterns. They volunteer at wild life refuges where they are able to stay free in their RV in exchange for working three days per week at the refuge. After listening to all their stories about where they traveled in their RV for 16 years and their birding expeditions, it made me realize that the world is your canvas and it is up to you to find out what's out there.

73. Ham radio club – one of my rollerblading friends is actively involved in the ham radio network and emergency response communication. You would be surprised as to how many people are involved in ham radio. On my cruise I met a German man talking about his ham radio and across the table from him was an Australian doing the same thing. They instantly hit it off talking about their equipment and the people they talked to from all over the world. Being a ham, you develop friends in distant lands that you can go visit.

74. **Short film production** - is an art form that few people think of. At the Wanee music festival in northern Florida, I interviewed a man between band changes that was a retired builder. When I asked him what he did for fun in retirement, he told me that he teaches photography at the art institute and has also won an award for short film production. He likes the creativity of writing and putting a short film together. He said that he was creative as a builder and short film production and photography allowed him to stay creative.

75. **How about working part time?** - I knew a lady that retired with her engineer husband to Florida. In retirement she decided to become a real estate agent specializing in high rise buildings close to where she lived. She moved from a 5 bedroom home up north to a spacious 1 bedroom condo downtown. When I asked her why such a drastic change, she said that she had lots of kids and relatives and did not want to be a bed and breakfast place for everyone coming down in the winter to visit. A beautiful Hilton hotel was just down the street so they could see each other as much as they wanted. The 1,050 square foot one bedroom condo was easy to take care of and big enough for both of them. To keep herself occupied, she thought that being a realtor and meeting all kinds of interesting people moving to Florida would be a lot of fun. She absolutely loved her retirement job. She enjoyed being socially engaged talking to new people and also making some money at the same time. Her husband was happy just playing baseball, monitoring their investments and going to cultural events. He was glad that she found something fulfilling to do in retirement. The arrangement worked for both of them. On my transatlantic voyage I met Andy at the breakfast table. The man looked 68 years old. He told me "as a human species we were bred to work" "what else can you do in an 8 hour day" he had worked in manufacturing as a mechanical engineer, lived in St Petersburg, Florida, lake Tahoe and now lives in Las Vegas selling real estate part time. He likes to work "I drive around in my golf cart showing people plots of land and now and then they write me a check, life is good" "I am 87 years old". He was an amazing man to talk to, fit, sharp and full of energy. I couldn't believe he was 87, he was in such good shape.

New research at the university in Melbourne Australia showed that working 25-30 hours per week sharpens your cognitive skills. The chapter on the mind explains memory stimulation in more detail

On a morning walk I saw an older gentleman in his late 70's carefully masking the decorative shutters on a six unit apartment building. I asked him "do you own this building" he said "yes I do" "do you want to sell it? He stood there and thought and shook his head "no" and then added "then I would have nothing to do". He felt that he needed to get out and do something on a regular basis to stay involved. it also probably kept him in a better mood and gave him a reason to get out of the house. There are many ways to work part time and some people like rehabbing or managing real estate.

CHAPTER 7

Clean Out/Detoxify Your Body

Imagine living in a house for forty, fifty, sixty, or seventy years. **How much junk do you accumulate?** Are you running out of storage space? Can you find anything you want at a moment's notice? Do you buy things over, and over, and over again because you forgot where you put them? Your internal body has the same problem.

Many years ago I was looking for a house in St Petersburg Florida. Since I lived in Atlanta at that time, I had a realtor pre select houses for me with certain criteria such as sunset views, a sailboat boat slip and so on. One day I received a call from my realtor and she said "A house that meets your criteria just came on the market". I flew down the next morning, looked at the house, and immediately offered the seller full price since the house met my criteria. As the realtor was filling out the paper work she said "the house is in a deed restricted community" I said what is that? She said basic rules like keeping your grass cut, bushes trimmed and so on in order to maintain the value of the neighborhood. Since I had no experience with deed restrictions, it seemed reasonable at the time. The deed restriction rules were handed to me after the closing. They became very real to me when I started getting deed restriction violation letters. I became very annoyed and stressed out with all the nit picking.

One of the most frequent deed restriction violation letters that I get was for having a dirty white tile roof. These letters come about every two years and I have to have the entire roof pressure washed. If I did not correct the violation within a month, I may get a more forceful letter from an attorney or be taken to court. One of the most aggravating violations came after my seawall collapsed. As I was dealing with trying to salvage my property and getting a new seawall built, I get a letter for illegally dumping dirt into the canal and silting up the waterway for other boaters. After the seawall was built, I had to hire a company to vacuum out the extra dirt in front of my seawall, an expensive process.

You are probably wondering how the deed restrictions relate to toxins that we unknowingly ingest. Those environmental toxins may make us sick or weaken our immune system.

How does a roof on the water in Florida get dirty and develop mold. Pollutants are in the air, they fall on the roof, the humidity and constant rain turns those pollutants into mold that creeps into the cracks and crevices of the tile roof. Before you know it, the roof starts looking greyer and greyer. As a homeowner you don't notice it, but the deed restriction watchdogs do and send you that nasty letter.

The pollutants on the roof are the same as the toxins in the food that we eat or the water or the air that we breathe. It only takes 2 years for my roof to get moldy and look bad. With the pollutants we are exposed to on a daily basis, our body will be just as bad. If you look at autopsied lungs of smokers, their lungs look grey and mottled just like my dirty roof. How about the internal components of our cells such as the mitochondria, the powerhouses of our cells. Are they functioning at their optimum capacity? Digested toxins are stored in our fat cells, the more fat cells you have, the greater are your chances of having a lot of potential carcinogens. Obesity is associated with a greater risk of cancer.

Over time your body becomes so cluttered with toxins that it starts to self-destruct. Those unknown toxins, like the molds on my roof, come from the air, the foods you eat, the chemicals, additives and preservatives in the food. The toxins on my roof come from the pollutants in the environment just like the toxins in our body.

We have no idea what's in our food, things we touch, in the air we breathe, or in the water we drink. Do we?

In New Mexico PFAS, the "forever chemicals", have been found in water sources. Most of those chemicals were downstream of major urban developments in the Rio Grande River. The studies were done by the US Geological survey and by the state's environmental agency, after the contaminants were discovered at military facilities. These PFAS, short name for perfluoroalkyl and polyfluoroalkyl chemicals are called forever substances because they do not decay in the environment and also stay circulating in our bodies. We have no way of getting rid of these chemicals. These chemicals are toxins, an immune hazard, associated with human cancer.

This is just one of the most recent examples of Toxins that we know nothing about that exist in our environment. There are many other potential toxins. According to Chemical and Engineering news published by the American Chemical society, the EPA, the environmental protection agency, has a list of 85,000 chemicals. There are an estimated 21 billion pounds of toxic chemicals released into our atmosphere by industry worldwide.

If you have trouble losing weight, you may by be a victim of the Obesogenics. Obesogenics are chemicals that affect human hormones and affect the way our bodies process and store fats. They are chemicals in our environment that cause us to gain weight such as BPA found in plastic water bottles and food containers and PFAS the forever chemical that take a long time to grade. These chemicals are found in food packaging, cleaning products, water-resistant fabric, nonstick cookware, shampoos, nail polish, eye makeup, stain resistant coatings on carpets, furniture, fabrics, grease resistant paper, umbrellas, tents, processed meats, sports drinks, chips etc.

What about micro and Nano plastics? Nano plastics are very small plastic particles that we ingest in our food. These plastic particles are so small that they can get into our cell membrane and cause toxic effects that we are just beginning to study. Studies on cadavers' brains have found an increasing amount of Nano plastics. It is estimated that there is a spoonful of Nano plastics in our brains. The amount of Nano plastics in our bodies is increasing as more animals are injecting plastics in their food sources and we are eating those animals.

All of us get thermal printed receipts from stores every day. Did you know that the thermal paper is coated with BPA or chemically related BPS and BPF? These chemicals are absorbed through the skin on our fingers and react with our hormonal system. They are endocrine disrupters especially of concern to women of child bearing age, pregnant or nursing women, teenagers and even the elderly. These chemicals can imitate our bodies own hormones and have undesirable consequences. According to studies done in Europe and Japan, they apparently mimic estrogen and how cells respond to natural estrogens. In animal studies BPA was linked to obesity, cancer and reproductive problems. In humans BPA has been associated with increased risk of diabetes and heart disease.

Isn't it sad that something as inconsequential as a thermal grocery store receipt may harm us? How about chemical compounds released in all the plastic containers that we microwave in? It might be safer not to touch those receipts and microwave in glass or lead free ceramic containers. A PhD friend of mine only uses stainless water bottles on his bicycle to prevent possible plastic leaching of chemicals. Another doctor friend of mine, who is a pathologist, has the receipts put in the grocery bag so she doesn't have to touch them.

Our Hormones are being replaced by unnatural chemicals that mimic hormones but do not do the same thing. To illustrate the danger that certain chemicals have on our finely tuned "dance of the hormones" think of a locks and keys. Each lock has a specific key that unlocks it. Some keys fit into several keyholes but they do not unlock the doors. The key may be made from a similar blank, but the pattern of ridges on the key is different so it fits in the lock but doesn't open the door.

Synthetic chemicals are like blank keys that may fit in the lock but cannot open the door.

If a lock has a key in it that doesn't open the door can the correct key be inserted on top of that key to open that door? No it cannot. Your room stays locked and you can't do anything with what's inside of that door. If it's a car, you can't drive the car. If you are a mechanic, you cannot unlock your tool box to repair a car. If it's your pantry, you cannot go in and get the ingredients to cook or bake can you?

Maybe that's why young ladies cannot get pregnant because the keyholes are full of useless synthetic estrogen keys? Maybe that's why we get cancer because the keyholes have blank keys in them and our immune repair system keys cannot get in and fix our bodies.

Food for Thought: It took millions of years of evolution for our bodies to adapt to the foods we eat. The plants and other food sources evolved with us at the same pace and our bodies learned how to use them for fuel and adapt to them. Suddenly in the 21st century we have thousands of chemicals thrown at us that we did not have time to adapt to, or be able to detoxify. How do you expect our immune system to adapt to so many synthetic products in our food chain in such a short time? It is all too fast and all very dangerous. **Our foods have become our poisons.** Think about this for a while.

In the late 1990's I saw a report about trans fatty acids on prime time national news. The headline was to the effect "The fats you eat may be killing you". It was a catchy headline, so I hung around listening to the main report, and it was about trans fatty acids and hydrogenated oils.

Trans fatty acids and hydrogenated oils are used throughout the processed food industry to preserve flavors in food and keep it from spoiling. **Experts say these trans fatty acids may be clogging your arteries** and may be one of the leading causes of the high incidence of cardiovascular disease and arteriosclerosis.

See, these things are not really natural, so the body has no effective way of eliminating them or dealing with them. As we were developing through the millions of years, our bodies developed to accommodate common things found in nature, animal fats, vegetables, proteins, carbohydrates, trace minerals, vitamins, and so forth. **Our bodies did not evolve to process the hundred thousand chemicals we are exposed to on a continuous basis. These things are man-made.**

The FDA finally banned the use of trans fatty acids in 2018. It took a lawsuit and overwhelming evidence for them to act. Why did it take so long? For how many years have you been eating trans fatty acids?

The interesting thing is that cardiovascular disease is still the number one killer. There must be many other chemicals in our food doing the same damage.

How about white bread? Is the FDA finally going to do something about it? Most of you are wondering what I am talking about. In order to have white bread the grain has to be bleached with either Chlorine or other chemicals. This bleaching process destroys many vitamins and nutrients naturally occurring and potentially adds alloxan, a byproduct of the bleaching process. Alloxan is used in laboratory animals to induce diabetes. The bleaching process also allows more sugar to be added to the bread. With the huge rise of diabetes in this country does eating bleached white bread make sense? The use of chlorine, bromates, and peroxides is banned in the European Union.

If you think that eating bleached bread is bad, how about eating plastic. A plastic material called azodicarbonamide (ADA) has been reported to be in 500 foods. It makes bread and pastries spongy, that's why it is also used in flip flops and exercise Matts. The thought of eating my flip flops makes me cringe.

What is even scarier are the plastics in the ocean. If you have ever seen photos of miles and miles of plastics floating in the oceans you would have gotten sick. I have seen piles of plastics on the Amazon River, on Asian rivers, on the beaches of Africa and plastics floating in the oceans. In sections of Africa, clean water is sold in small plastic pouches which are discarded, ending up in the oceans and on the beaches. Those plastics are eventually broken down into micro plastics. Those micro plastics are ingested by the plankton.

Small fish eat the plankton and bigger fish eat the small fish. By the time we eat fish, chances are that you are ingesting plastics that were passed up in the food chain.

Have you ever thought about coffee? Most of us drink this beverage every morning. Do you know if the coffee beans have been sprayed with pesticides? Did you know that coffee plants have up to 250 pounds of pesticides per acre sprayed on them? We may be grinding and boiling those pesticides right into our bodies. True, there may be some high end mountain grown coffee beans out there where pesticide machines can't reach, but most of us are totally unaware of which beans are pesticide free since most are imported. Look to see if the coffee is certified organic, labeled sustainable or grown traditionally, before pesticides/fungicides were invented. Coffee is cardio protective and helps reduce the incidence of type 2 diabetes according to newest research. Two to five cups of coffee appear to be OK according to the new US dietary guidelines.

The fruits and vegetables we eat are all sprayed to prevent bugs and fungi from eating them. What effect are those pesticides having on our bodies? Even if we wash our fruits and vegetables thoroughly the small quantities absorbed through their skin may still be enough to cause chronic diseases 10 or 40 years from now because they are slowly accumulated in our system. "Buyer beware", because the food that we consume may slowly be destroying us and specific food that we fail to consume may be needed to protect us from those environmental adulterated food toxins.

Over the last fifty to sixty years, big business, primarily the food and biochemical industries, have figured out how to make things taste good, look good and last forever. They also created **GMO's** – genetically modified foods. In their quest for economic gain, **they didn't take into consideration the long term effects of these chemical substances and altered genes on our health.** It's all about yield per acre (hector) money and profit.

Through our industrialized society, millions of tons of **toxic waste** are created but there is nowhere to put it. In 1998 it was reported that the government allowed this toxic waste residue from large manufacturing companies and smoldering plants to be ground up, **mixed into fertilizers**, and spread upon our soil within certain thresholds. These toxins are absorbed by the plants along with the fertilizer, passed on through the food chain, and we, as the ultimate consumers of the food chain, **absorb them in our bodies**. Pressure treated wood has enough toxins in it, such as Arsenic, to be considered a hazard. Did you know that it was excluded from the hazardous waste law? In 1994 it was discontinues for residential use. How about all the pressure treated wood we are exposed to that was manufactured from 1940 to 2004?

You had no idea they were doing that, did you? Very few people do. These chemicals sludge up your system so severely that it doesn't function properly. A sludge infested body is more susceptible to a variety of ailments.

You have been living in your body for fifty, sixty, seventy or eighty years. That's a long time for junk to accumulate and clog up your biological system. You accumulate this junk through the foods you eat and air you breathe. **Probably the most recognizable form of clogging is cardiovascular disease**. Years and years of accumulations of bad sugars, processed fats, and genetically altered fats combined with other toxic elements in our food, air, and environment slowly clog up the system. **Eventually, the system breaks down and develops obstruction of the blood supply to major organs.**

When that obstruction occurs in the heart, we get restriction of blood flow and oxygenation and nutrients to the heart muscle causing heart stress. If enough damage occurs, the heart attack we get leads to total heart failure and our demise.

Modern medicine's solution to that problem is to insert a stent or bypass two to three inches of a blood vessel with a vein grafted from your leg. **That vein is not as strong as the original vessel it replaces and it eventually also clogs up.**

The bypass procedure is nothing more than **an expensive Band-Aid for an emergency treatment. It does not cure the disease.** It does make people feel better and it does increase blood supply to certain sections of the heart for a limited time.

Did you ever ask yourself, **"What about the other seventy five million miles of blood vessels that I have in my body? What's happening to them and the rest of my organ systems and my brain? Are they getting enough blood supply and nutrition?"**

The answer is obvious. **If it is obstructing your heart, it is obstructing the rest of your system**.

How about less obvious clogging systems, which occur in Alzheimer's disease or other chronic ailments that can eventually lead to abnormal cell functions and ultimately our death. In **Alzheimer's disease**, researchers have found higher concentrations of aluminum, as well as a sludge-type material, beta amyloid the residue of dead nerve cells, neurofibrillary tangles, and abnormal accumulation of Tau protein and neuro inflammation. Loss of microcirculation in our brains may be another culprit in dementias.

This sludge-type material eventually clogs up the cell mechanisms so the nerve cells cannot function properly and communicate. After a while, they become so inundated with the garbage that has been deposited over the years they die.

As neurons die, you gradually lose the ability to think. How sad, spending a lifetime achieving goals, being active, relishing your children and grandchildren, not to be able to enjoy your old age. By the way, what do you have when you get older? You have your memories. When your memories are gone, as has occurred in former president Ronald Reagan, you can't even enjoy your past achievements in old age. **A part of your life has been robbed**.

What about cancer and other chronic degenerative conditions? Can you catch cancer from someone else as they sneeze at you? Can you catch cancer from a cut that you get on a broken piece of glass? Can you catch cancer when you have a cold?

Cancer is a failure of your body to regulate itself, a failure in the immune system. Cells of the primary site just keep on replicating themselves. It's going back to the same mechanism that caused your cardiovascular disease, caused your Alzheimer's disease, and causes a lot of other chronic conditions. It is a sludging up of your system with junk that impedes your auto repair processes. Cells just keep on proliferating out of control. **It is a failure of your immune system to recognize the cancer cells and keep you healthy.**

You slowly becomes clogging up and your biological system becomes overwhelmed with unnatural junk. Over time, the body just can't handle it and it starts functioning abnormally.

The body does not repair itself properly or the cells continue to replicate themselves unchecked until they kill you, which is exactly what happens in cancer.

The checks and balances are lost because there is so much junk built up in your system. The more chemicals you inject through processed foods and additives, the greater your chances of developing a chronic disease your body can't handle because there is too much sludge clogging up your natural reparative mechanisms.

The modern agricultural food business, including the fast food industry, has produced food that is loaded with high fructose corn syrup and devoid of essential nutrients. Modern foods are devoid of vitamins and minerals, and loaded with chemical additives, preservatives, and unnatural fats. Poor quality foods have caused more than half of the United States population to be obese and at the same time nutritionally starved.

This greed for profit in **our food industry has created a time bomb** in our population that will eventually lead to a slew of chronic degenerative diseases, which will make the quality of our lives miserable.

There is a remedy: Clean out the body and gives it pure and nutrient-laden foods, necessary supplements, and adequate amounts of pure, clean, unadulterated water, essential for cleansing our body, increasing the function of our kidneys, and normalizing our cellular fluids, intra and extracellular. You want to give your liver, the main detoxifying organ, a rest.

Detoxification is the removal or toxic substances from our body. It is primarily done by the liver but other organs such as the kidneys, the lymph system, our skin, lungs also act as detoxifies. You have heard of alcohol detox, drug detox, poison antidotes, narcotics overdose antidotes and dialysis. Dialysis is detoxification because your kidneys are not doing their job anymore filtering out toxins. If your liver fails, you need a transplant. For prescription drug detoxification the body uses a detox program called the xenobiotic mechanism which involves a series of oxidase reactions to neutralize the drug. There is detoxification going on all the time in your body. So, what can you do to help that process along?

The first thing you do is limit depositing toxic chemicals in your body and on your body. Unhealthy chemicals that cause your body to break down. Yes, I know. Fatty foods, fries, greasy chicken, processed foods, all kinds of snack food, and ready-to-eat meals are things you enjoy. Of course, they are. **They are engineered to taste good, look good, and smell good. They are not necessarily engineered to be healthy.**

You may enjoy eating them, but **consider the long-term consequences.** The first thing you need to do is limit what you take in. More about that will be discussed in a later chapter.

The next thing you have to do, as the title of this chapter says, is clean your system out**. Detoxify yourself**. You see, once your body gets rid of a large portion of the stored toxins and sludge that was accumulated over a long period of time, it will be more organized. The biological processes will work better, the chemical interactions, digestion, repair mechanisms they will all function at a more optimal capacity thereby decreasing your chances of developing these chronic debilitating diseases, such as adult onset diabetes, cancer, cardiovascular disease, Alzheimer's disease, and so on. **If your body works at peak efficiency, there is less chance of biological breakdown**, which causes a lot of these disease processes. The less stress you put on the system, the better it will work. Just think of work stress, emotional stress, and financial stress. If there is enough stress on the system, eventually something has to give. You want to limit your chemical stress, psychological stress and environmental stress as much as possible to prevent that break down.

There are numerous ways one can detoxify oneself. One of the oldest ways of detoxification is **sweating**. It is a tradition that started in Europe, Turkey, and the Middle East when people used saunas to induce perspiration. The theory was that by sweating, toxins can be eliminated through the skin's pores, allowing the body to purify itself. Sweating **is a very effective way to rid the body of excess waste through your skin.**

The second largest organ in our body is our skin, the vascular system is the largest. The skin is very efficient in eliminating endogenous toxic compounds along with fluids from the body. Without skin, we would die. A good example is people whose skin has been severely burned over large portions of their bodies. With so much of their skin damaged, they easily succumb to infections and die.

Skin is also a semi-permeable membrane. Certain substances pass right through it. Therefore, **external toxins** we touch or are exposed to in the air are absorbed by our skin and can poison us slowly. Medications are given through the skin through patches and creams.

Just as the skin absorbs toxins, the skin can excrete toxins. Taking **saunas or steam baths** has been a popular method of detoxification throughout the centuries and is currently used extensively throughout the world. In Europe people go to spas so they can stay healthy. They will say "I feel better afterward".

Another way of obtaining similar benefits is by exercising to the point that you **sweat**. The type of exercise and duration of exercise will be addressed in a later chapter.

Unlike exercising to produce sweat, sauna sweating requires no effort. You just sit there and let your metabolism do the work. The body tries to cool itself because of the excess heat, and it does that by perspiring. As the body perspires, toxins are released through the pores. Another option is to move to Florida and sweat in the summer humidity.

There are a number of **herbal teas** that have been used for detoxification as well. You can find many of them in the health stores. **Ginseng** is one of the most common detoxification agents. **Chamomile** tea, used in Europe quite a bit, is another. **Ginkgo biloba** has also become popular. Drinking eight to ten glasses of pure water per day is a simple way to clean out your system.

Herbal teas are even being used to pass drug tests. If you look on the Internet, you'll find several companies that have various herbal tea products that cause you to urinate and detoxify any drug residue left in your body, allowing people to pass drug tests. As noted in the above examples, **herbs are potent detoxifying agents.** At Northwestern University researchers found that brewed tea leaves absorb heavy metals. Heavy metal ions stick to the surface of the tea leaves.

For a zinger of a detoxifying tea, you may try the **Garlic – Ginger tea.** It consists of a bulb of crushed garlic, a thinly sliced lemon, a handful of thinly sliced ginger, a pinch or two of turmeric, cayenne pepper and honey. The garlic, ginger and turmeric are boiled for an hour in about a liter or quart of water. After boiling add the sliced lemon and a pinch of cayenne pepper (do not touch the pepper with your fingers or rub your eyes) and let it sit 20min. You can add some more water and then strain the contents for the tea. Add honey while hot 1-2 teaspoons before drinking. You can refrigerate and reheat the tea adding honey each time before drinking. You may be surprised how you feel afterwards. You may have fewer colds in the flu season or when flying in planes.

My niece in Poland uses a mixture of garlic, horseradish, ginger and apple cider vinegar in water to fight colds and boost the immune system.

Fasting is one form of detoxification and cleansing that is often ignored. **Our bodies were designed to have periods of starvation.** These periods of starvation are part of our nutritional cycle. Throughout the millions of years of human development, there never existed a period of time as we have today when food was so plentiful.

The body adapted to storing as many nutrients as possible in our fat cells when there was plenty and to utilize those nutrients in periods of food deficiency. A newly discovered protein switch called **mTOR** is responsible for turning on our anabolic cycle, where we store fat derived from sugar in fat cells. The metabolic syndrome diseases such as hypertension and type 2 diabetes are a result of this switch being constantly on. When this switch is turned off our body goes into catabolism by first using up the glycogen stores for energy and then burning fats. Fasting turns off the mTOR switch and the body goes into a conservation protective mode. It tries to be as efficient as possible protecting its organs and removing inflammatory toxins that it accumulated in the anabolic cycle.

This cycle of feast and famine has been a normal cycle in our human evolutionary development. This cycle also played an important component in **ridding our bodies of unnecessary toxins that accumulated in the plentiful cycle**. However, with the abundance and excess of food, this normal cleansing phase has not had a chance to kick in, and **we have continuously stored toxins absorbed through our food chain, and through our skin and lungs, without a chance to refresh ourselves.**

Fasting has been used throughout the centuries as a method to purify the body. There are numerous **biblical references to fasting** going back thousands of years. Many religions have used fasting as a purification before their major holidays. It was not just self-sacrifice for which fasting was used. Fasting was recognized as a means of **cleansing the body of impurities.**

A number of years ago, when I was studying for my first doctorate, I developed an interest in fasting and I read a well-documented book that broke down specifically the body's physiological effects to fasting.

When the body is not getting external energy from proteins, carbohydrates, or fats, it has to look internally for reserves. This internal approach mobilizes biochemical processes and **chemical reactions that are not normally used, because we live in a world of excess.**

This triggering of chemical reactions, which forces the body to utilize glycogen, fat, and even protein stores of fuel, mobilizes some of the stored impurities embedded in our fat cells. As the fat is burned for fuel, some of those impurities are excreted through the urinary system and skin.

Periodic fasts of one to three days are used routinely in European countries as cleansing mechanisms and allow the body's unused biochemical processes to function therefore providing us with alternate sources of fuel. When I did my last fast of 2.5 days, I drank sparkling water and occasionally added 1-2 oz. of gator aid or orange juice for electrolytes and flavor. I lost 7 lbs. and felt great. During my fast I walked 3 hours the second day and kept hydrated. When I started to eat, it was only a small amount of food and mostly fruits and vegetables with some protein. Your stomach shrinks so you feel full right away. Two days after fasting, I had a lot of energy without the desire to eat a lot of food.

On my world cruise, I fasted for 32 hours to get to my new target weight of 161 lbs. (73 kg). My goal was to reduce my set point from 163 lbs. to 161 lbs. The set point is where I allow my weight to fluctuate up or down by 2 pounds.

During the fast the hunger went away after 24 hours. I could have fasted longer but my weight was below my target weight and I was told that my breath smelled real bad. After 4 months cruising, I was 4 lbs. lighter than when I started.

If I gain 2 lbs., I reduce my food intake by skipping meals. If I lose 2 lbs. then I will increase my food intake. On the cruise I use a portable scale in ports and at home a balance bar doctors scale which has my previous weight on the slider. I weigh myself every few days. My college weight was 162 lbs. and my high school weight 155 lbs. I now maintain my weight closer to my high school weight.

Intermittent Fasting has become the new Fast. Researchers at several universities have started to study the effects of intermittent fasting on out physiology by doing controlled before and after blood work studies. The most popular intermittent fast is the 5:2 fast. For five days you eat normally and for 2 days you reduce your calorie intake to 600 calories if you are a man and 500 calories if you are a woman. The theory behind this intermittent fast is that it is protein sparing. You burn primarily glycogen and fat instead of muscle for energy. New research published in the "Annals of Internal Medicine", found that intermittent fasting is as good as calorie counting for weight loss. Subjects were able to keep weight off over a year. The people were not asked to restrict their calories, but by limiting eating to an 8 hour window, they ended up eating 400 fewer calories per day. The study showed that subjects were able to keep up the intermittent fasting habit for a year. This is important because it shows that intermittent fasting is a doable lifestyle and health style choice. The other benefit is that you look better.

Always ask your doctor if your health condition is able to tolerate a fast. With the rampant advent of diabetes and other health conditions, you may not be able to tolerate even an intermittent fast.

It is important to remember that **copious amounts of water are necessary when one undergoes a fasting program** since water is a key ingredient in many of the biochemical reactions to burn body stores of fuel.

I generally recommend at least **one-half to one gallon of water per day for my patients** and have seen mild bladder infections clear up with a gallon of water a day and some cranberry juice mixed in. Newer scientific research has shown that cranberry juice helps prevent bacteria from adhering to the bladder wall therefore reducing the incidence of infections. The studies did not find that once an infection has established itself that cranberry juice helps get rid of it, therefore making antibiotic drugs necessary.

We can auto-detoxify ourselves by avoiding alcohol and fructose based sugars, in order to rest the liver and pancreas, and by flushing out our systems with pure **osmotically-filtered or distilled water** in adequate amounts. We can assist the body in flushing itself on a daily basis, giving a continuous cleansing, the same way that daily bowel movements move digested waste out of our systems **so we don't absorb the harmful chemicals that are putrefying in our guts.**

Colonoscopies have become routine and help detect early colon cancers. They are recommended to be done by age 40 now, and every 10 years after. Colon cancer is one of the few preventable cancers if detected early in the pre-cancerous stage through colonoscopy.

Talking about our gut leads us to another form of detoxification, which has been used for a long period of time, **colonic irrigation**. Colonics do not sound pleasant. As a matter of fact, they sound repulsive. However**, Fleet enemas** have been a normal part of medical procedures for a long time for constipation and to cleanse the gut of fecal toxins that have been accumulating. **A colonic is a deeper form of intestinal cleansing.** The practitioner performing the procedure must be a licensed and certified health care provider that uses sterile equipment, so that there is no cross contamination from others. Probiotics may be a good idea afterwards to make sure you have adequate beneficial bacteria in your gut.

Many times there is inadequate intestinal motility to eliminate impacted particles or feces that after a while sit in little pockets and cause craters leading to, you guessed it, colon cancer or polyps, as well as overall illness, because the **byproducts of digestion are actually toxic**. The indoles and skatols that are produced, as well as other chemicals, are harmful to the body. **Chronic constipation or improper bowel motility can lead to chronic diseases**. A colonic is a process by which you lie on your side, draped, and a sterile cannula is inserted into your rectum. Warm water is circulated through your bowels and extracted. Any impacted or stagnant material is flushed out and eliminated, leaving you with a clean gut. It's not as awful as it sounds and is not painful. The reason that I informed you of colonics is because most people never heard of them. If you have impaction problems, colonics are an option to consider. Colonoscopy preps are another.

Other enemas have also been used to detoxify the gut; the purpose of me informing you about gut cleansing is to make you aware that the intestinal system and **the gut can be a source of auto-intoxication** and, therefore, needs to be regularly cleaned out. **Regular bowel movements are very important.** Prunes do a lot for bowel mobility and so does consuming roughage.

One of the main causes of colon cancer is the lack of movement of digested food through our gut, and the resultant prolonged exposure to toxins that need to be eliminated through our feces. Putrefied meat produces a lot of toxins.

The last topic I want to talk about regarding "cleaning it out" or detoxification is **chelation therapy**. The theory of chelation was invented in Europe at the turn of the twentieth century. As a matter of fact, Dr. Alfred Werner, a German-Swiss scientist, won a Nobel Prize in 1913 for inventing chelation. The German chemical industry had a heck of a time removing impurities from their chemicals, especially the dye industry. They had difficulty getting a pure color because of the calcium deposition, as well as other metal and mineral deposits that crept into their chemicals. They used Dr. Werner's invention to find the impurities and remove them from their substances so they would have the pure chemical that they needed.

Chelation uses a synthetic amino acid, **EDTA (ethylene diamine tetra-acetic acid)**, to **bind toxic metals** in a heterocyclic ring, a fancy term meaning it encircles the object and forces it to bind to it.

In humans, once the toxic metal or mineral is bound, **you pee it out—it's simple and effective.**

Chelation is used in many of our household goods. One of the most common is mayonnaise. EDTA keeps mayonnaise from going rancid by preventing oxidation, which causes rancidity. By using EDTA, the free radicals cannot destroy the mayonnaise as easily, thereby keeping it fresh. Otherwise, it would spoil within a matter of days. **It is a potent antioxidant**.

Chelation is also used in shower cleaners. Look at some of the major brands and you will see EDTA as one of the ingredients. It binds the shower scum and helps remove it from your shower walls.

In humans, **chelation was first used** in the 1950's for people suffering from **lead poisoning**, as in battery plants in Detroit, Michigan. Dr. Norman Clark at Providence Hospital in Detroit, used chelation for the first time **to detoxify heavy metals** from workers exposed to lead, who suffered from numerous neurological conditions due to lead toxicity. After administering intravenous chelation, those workers got well and their neurological conditions improved.

When Dr. Clark reported his beneficial effects with battery plant workers, chelation caught on for the treatment of heavy metal poisoning. **The U.S. Government started using it to treat painters who painted the bottoms of ships with lead paint**. Many ship painters developed severe neurological problems due to the heavy metal toxicity. With chelation therapy, those patients also got better.

As chelation started to be used more and more for toxic metal poisoning, and it is still the treatment of choice for children with lead toxicity from lead paint, doctors started noticing **other beneficial effects** they had not expected. One of the most prominent was **circulatory** effects. Patients who had symptoms of **arteriosclerotic disease, such as chest pain, intermittent claudication, decreased energy**, and so forth, improved, and reported less chest pains, increased ability to walk and increased energy.

Because of those observations, doctors started using chelation for circulatory problems. Currently, over a million people have received chelation therapy for all kinds of conditions ranging from **ulcerations and gangrene of the feet due to diabetes, neuropathy, impaired circulation in the legs, heart, and brain, memory loss, decreased energy, heavy metal toxicity, and as a preventative measure**. I have noticed remarkable results in a lot of my patients who have had chelation therapy at the chelation medical centers.

It appears that **when the toxins** in our food chain and our environment that have been impeding our body chemical repair and regulatory cycles, **are removed, the body functions better. I have seen patients' memory improve**. After chelation therapy, patients who had to write sticky notes all over the place to remember things to do, no longer needed those reminders. I have seen patients' **diabetic neuropathy improve**. I have seen **ulcerations improve**. Notably, I see a marked **increase in energy** in a lot of my patients and **a willingness to do more and be active in life**, even into their old age. One of the more remarkable things I have seen is that patients, even those who have had a stroke, become more alert in terms of their environment. They develop an interest in things whereas before, they were content to not do much of anything. These are anecdotal findings reported by relatives, that have not been scientifically tested, but, nevertheless worth mentioning.

Chelation therapy is received intravenously. In my chelation centers patients reclined in comfortable chairs and could read, nap, eat, drink or chat with other patients while the infusion flowed into their veins.

Chelation therapy is not only the intravenous administration of a synthetic amino acid, EDTA, it **also involves administration of certain vitamins concurrently.** Patients receive B vitamins, as well as vitamin C, in their IV drip and are given multiminerals and multivitamins to supplement any trace elements that are lost that are necessary to the body. Patients are also **instructed in dietary changes, as well as exercise regimens** to go along with their chelation therapy.

Taking all of that into consideration, not all patients follow the recommendations. Yet even those who get only the intravenous chelation drip have had remarkable improvements based upon my clinical observations. Numerous other studies have concurred with those observations. Some of those studies will be referenced later in this book.

Since the first edition of this book was written in 2000, a great deal of research has been done in chelation therapy. The National Center for Complementary and Alternative Medicine, a division of the **NIH** (National Institute of Health**)**, began a Trial to Assess Chelation Therapy (TACT) in 2003 due to pressure from physicians administering chelation and from patients. The trial was to study the validity of chelation for treating conditions other than heavy metal poisoning. The trial was also supported by the American College of Cardiology. Alternative minded physicians who were certified to administer chelation therapy by ACAM (the American College for the Advancement of Medicine) were observing a variety of benefits in their patients that needed to be further investigated on a controlled basis.

The study started in 2003 with final results being published November 2012 long after the first edition of this book was published. The authors concluded that disodium EDTA chelation "modestly" reduced the risk of adverse cardiovascular outcomes among stable patients with a history of myocardial infarction. The study also showed **a "marked" reduction in cardiovascular events in diabetic patients treated with EDTA chelation.** An editorial published in **the Journal of the American Medical Association** said that "the study findings may provide novel hypotheses that merit further evaluation to help understand the pathophysiology of secondary prevention of vascular disease."

What surprised me was the JAMA editorial, since there has been so much criticism of chelation for conditions other than heavy metal toxicity in the past. The words "marked" reduction in cardiovascular events in diabetics were significant to me since I found peripheral small vessel benefits in my patients where the tingling in their feet disappeared and normal color returned to their feet. These were incidental benefits that patients told me and have not been specifically studied in a controlled trial. Patients undergoing EDTA chelation therapy are also advised to follow healthy lifestyle choices such as avoid sugars and saturated fats, eat a lot of fruits and vegetables, increase exercise and maintain proper weight.

Use your own judgement, do your own research since there are differences of opinion in this treatment for conditions other than heavy metal poisoning. I included chelation therapy in the detoxifying chapter because it does detoxify and everyone agrees on that.

Most doctors have limited knowledge about the benefits of chelation or about this major study.

So let's tie all this together. I began this chapter with a house that gradually became cluttered with stuff that you can't find when you need it. That stuff made your house uninhabitable because you kept on buying more stuff to replace the stuff you can't find. That stuff is similar to the accumulation of toxins in our body making it uninhabitable.

We **constantly eat foods**, either in restaurants where the food was cooked in **aluminum pans** and the aluminum, which is a **neurotoxin**, is absorbed in the food and eventually deposited in our brains and other tissues, as well as thousands and **thousands of chemicals, hormones, antibiotics and additives added to our food.** They make food grow faster, look good, and last longer. We inadvertently eat and store those chemicals in our house, our body.

We eat food because it looks good, tastes good, smells good gives us a pleasant gastronomical experience. On the world cruise they have special food nights, today we had seafood extravaganza lunch buffet, the other day we had a French night and the week before we had a German night. Each of those specialty food nights feature foods from specific countries loaded with calories. The escargot plate was flooded with butter. All the above foods were yummy, but, **the adulteration of foods in our food chain is slowly toxifying us.**

The chemical load and toxic metal load that is placed upon us gradually **wears down our immune systems** to the point where our resistance is very low and any abnormal stressor to our systems can set off a chronic degenerative condition. Did you ever ask yourself, with all the miracles of medicine, **why is**

cardiovascular disease the number one killer and cancer the number two killer in the United States?

President Richard Nixon declared the war on cancer on December 23, 1971 and things just keep on getting worse.

All of these conditions are self-induced by things we voluntarily store in our bodies, such as cancer-forming chemicals from cigarette smoking, or even artificial sweeteners? **We don't know the long-term effects on our bodies through involuntary storage of chemicals from all the processed food we eat on a daily basis.**

When was the last time you **read the labels of all the foods** you are eating? Do you know what all the chemical names are that are on that label? Do you know what they are used for? Do you know how they are stored in the body or excreted from the body? Do you know what secondary reactions they may have to impede our body from working properly? You don't.

You just blindly believe that everything the biochemical food technology complex industry (whose primary motive is profit) puts into our foods is safe. Well, I have news for you.

It isn't safe. Over a long time **it may have a very deleterious effect on your health and cause you to become susceptible to many** degenerative conditions that slowly rob you of your quality of life.

We all want to be active, energetic, mentally alert, and healthy when we grow older. We want to be able to enjoy the fruits of our labor. However, with the **gradual poisoning of our bodies**, that dream may not be obtainable.

Where is my proof? My proof is the number one and number two killers in the USA, Heart Disease and Cancer. They are not infectious diseases. They are **self-induced diseases,** either voluntarily or involuntarily, by deposits placed in your body by environmental exposure to processed foods and other pollutants. **Other countries and civilizations that do not eat the same types of foods we eat, do not have the same chronic diseases or cancers that we do.**

They develop our diseases when they start eating our food.

Remember, **garbage in equals garbage out**. If you put in too much garbage willingly or unwillingly, you are going to have **an immunologically frail body, rich in calories, poor in nutrients and loaded with toxins**. We do not want to be like the Falcons in Shenandoah National Park, slowly becoming extinct. **Detoxification and cleaning out your body is one of the secrets of healthy aging.** If you want a nice looking house, clean out the clutter.

CHAPTER 8
Nutrients

This section has been used by readers as a reference.

For detailed chapters on "Vitamins, Minerals, Herbs and Anti-Oxidants" and "Hormones" please read my previous book "Happy Life Healthy Aging". My previous book went into great detail in explaining hormones, vitamins, minerals, trace minerals and other nutrients as to how they functioned. This chapter is designed to give you the basics. Most people do not need to know exactly how all the components of a car work in order to drive it.

Hippocrates said "Let food be thy medicine and let medicine be thy food". You have to ask yourself **is the food we eat today really food?**

Fruits, vegetables and dietary choices are important. This chapter nudges you towards making wiser choices in what you eat. It is good to know why you are doing something instead of just taking some magic pill that you know nothing about. Every human body is slightly different. This is the only body that we have, so we better make sure we give it the best building blocks possible in order for it to grow healthy and repair itself when things go wrong.

Currently our ship is on Null Island. "0" Latitude and "0" Longitude. It is your duty to find out where that is.

During my world voyage we had a guest presenter that talked about how technology has changed our lives. In a morning chat session she was asked about her previous life before she became a guest presenter. It turned out that she was trained as a physiotherapist in England as well as a nutritionist. She was also a personal trainer to famous corporate executives and movie stars in Hong Kong for 20 years at various private clubs. This lady was in her 70s and very fit. Someone in the chat session audience asked her "which is more important diet or exercise", without hesitation she answered "diet, because it is the building block of everything"

As you will see in this chapter, **diet is important in building a strong house but exercise keeps everything within that house working**. A house has a lot more than just the building blocks, a house has integrated systems that talk to one another and are interdependent. Your refrigerator needs electricity in order to work just like your body. You need to maintain that house on a regular basis or else things fall apart. Sandy, the fitness instructor on my world cruise would say "if it hurts, replace it". With nutrients we can replace cells, our building blocks, with higher quality building blocks. We chose the type of building blocks we use by making wise dietary choices.

After listening to Shenandoah National Park Rangers give their talks, I noticed that topics they covered in Nature had direct implications to this book.

Shenandoah National Park in Virginia used to have Peregrine Falcons. Over a dozen years they slowly disappeared from the park and no one knew why.

After prolonged study, it was determined that the DDT sprayed crops eaten by insects and then eaten by small birds who in turn were eaten by the falcons, was the culprit. The DDT infested prey of the Falcons caused their egg shells to be thin and break easily. Without strong egg shells the young hatching chicks could not survive because they broke while being laid or due to the elements. No new Falcons were born and the species became extinct in the park.

After DDT was banned, new falcons were introduced into the park. According to the park rangers, only one pair so far has stayed and reproduced with its offspring staying in the park. It's a lot harder to get something back after you lose it. The same is true with our health. (I pointed that out in the Physical Activity and Exercise chapter)

This is a perfect example of harmful chemicals that we do not know about, that are in our food. Throughout my RV travels I would see many pesticide spray tractors with large booms on either side spraying the crops, also crop duster airplanes buzzing overhead. I couldn't help but wonder how this spraying might be affecting our future generations? Did you ever wonder why "Low T" has become such a big business? Are men really producing less testosterone nowadays? Through the science of epigenetics how is this going to affect our great, great, grandchildren? The food we eat today does have an effect on future generations. That research was done in Scandinavia where they kept accurate records of past generations diets.

This chapter on Dietary choices is important because it gives you guidelines on how to select healthy foods that may affect your health in the future.

As I watched a program on PBS about the damming of Little Colorado River to make Lake Powell I noticed similarities in the ecological changes that have occurred to that river and its habitats and what happens to the human body.

You see, the scientists for the Department of Natural Resources had only looked at the Little Colorado and its course through the Grand Canyon. What would happen to the river upstream where the area was dammed up was their lone concern.

They gave no thought to the changes five miles, ten miles, or even fifty miles downstream. They didn't know that creation of a dam and alteration of the water flow would change the natural fish populations and their distributions. The scientists only started wondering about that when they noticed the native fish populations dying off, and fish not native to the region began to increase in numbers. On that PBS program, they admitted they had looked at the river as small segments instead of the one big entity it was; they failed to take note that a change upstream would affect the habitats of species a hundred miles downstream.

So they decided to push the system out of equilibrium a little bit further, and create a small flood, called the Grand Canyon flood, to see if they could change the environment back to its natural habitat. Well, guess what happened?

Large boulders eroded off the banks, entire beaches disappeared, new sediments appeared at other parts of the river, and the fish and wildlife species more or less tried to adapt to this temporary change in the water flow.

The scientists knew there would be erosion, after all, look at the Grand Canyon, a master example of the power of water reshaping landscape with its deep canyons and rainbow-colored vistas. At the end of their mini-flood experiment, the scientists marveled and said, **"Nature is not easily led or dominated."** It has resilience, but entire species of animals and plants can be totally wiped out just by changing the balanced equilibrium.

Just think of our colon, when we wipe out entire species of native organisms through excessive antibiotic use, the landscape is no longer the same. New organisms pop up that are not natural to our gut environment, and beneficial intestinal bacteria are annihilated. The intestinal organisms that make up our Bioderm are thrown out of balance. When the system is out of balance, certain organisms, such a C-dif can grow unchecked and rapidly kill us. My cousin died of C-dif rapid overgrowth 3 days after a "successful" elective heart surgery.

Water changed the Colorado River landscape forever, just as it is changing our biological equilibriums.

In the human body, we call this equilibrium **homeostasis, meaning maintaining things in balance**. Like the Little Colorado River's landscape, wildlife, and banks are influenced by the boulders rolling down with the river's force, along with the grasses, vegetation, and banks being altered. Our body reacts the same way to what we put through it.

The type of water we drink has a vast effect on every single chemical reaction that exists in our body. The more polluted and unnatural the water is, the greater will be the stress that eventually erodes our body and causes deep furrows like the Grand Canyon, and with time causes permanent scars affecting our biological equilibrium, like the altered shorelines and rapids caused by large boulder accumulations that create churning, swirling turbulence making it nearly impossible for anyone to navigate the river.

The debris we accumulate through our ingested liquids and foods makes it nearly impossible for our biological interactions to work properly or the blood to flow smoothly throughout our vessels. The intima, the innermost layer of our blood vessels gets damaged. This disrupting smooth vessel damage causes eddies, jetties, and rapids of its own eventually leading to arteriosclerosis and our demise through stroke, heart attack, or senility.

Yes, my ladies and gentlemen, **it all starts with the water.**

Our bodies are made up of between fifty and seventy percent water. If you have a lot of fat, it is closer to fifty percent; if you're lean, it's closer to seventy percent. Water is an essential component in every cell in our bodies.

Water is required for nutrient transfer to our cells. It is important for our brain cells to work, our lungs to work, and our entire absorption system of foods. Our muscles, including our heart, would stop working without adequate water. Because we lose water through respiration (breathing) and perspiration, as well as urination, we would survive only a few days without a constant supply.

One good thing is that the body constantly changes itself and you have a chance of rebuilding yourself every year. Did you know that your red blood cells only last about three months? That's right, you have all new oxygen carrying red blood cells every 90 days. You lose 50 million skin cells per day and develop a new gut lining every 10 days. I have read that your entire body recycles itself about every seven years. All these chemical reactions are dependent on water since water is the perfect solvent that allows us to transfer minerals and nutrients, as well as vitamins, into our cells. But all is not well in the water world.

Contamination with toxic chemicals, fertilizers, and additives have made our water dangerously polluted, to the point where it can interfere with our body's enzymatic pathways, as well as normal metabolism.

These interferences can cause massive stress on our body, which eventually wears down our repair mechanisms and we get catastrophic diseases, such as cancer, senility, cardiovascular disease, and so on. What are the plastic water bottles and Nano plastics doing to our water?

I read a report once that **one part per million of a toxic chemical**, of which we have many in our normal drinking water, produces **six-hundred-quadrillion toxic molecules**. That is 600, plus 15 zeros. That's a heck of a lot of toxic molecules that could be interfering with our normal cell function, eventually leading to cell death, abnormal replication, or just tired, worn-out cells that are tired of fighting these chemicals. Might that have something to do as to why we haven't been able to win the war on cancer?

When I went to Memorial University in Newfoundland to talk to the lead researcher in the Canadian Longevity Aging Study, I noticed that no one was there. What happened was that they shut that part of the university down for a day because of unacceptable high levels of Lead in the drinking water of several buildings, they were trying to find the source of this toxic heavy metal. Do you know what's in your water?

One interesting thing, substances such as chlorine and fluoride are added to water, which are known to cause major health problems. **Chlorine** is added to kill off dangerous bacteria. However, when chlorine is combined with organic substances, you end up with **chlorinated hydrocarbons, a toxin** to the body, which may cause hardening of the arteries, heart attacks, and other age-related diseases.

There is a book written by Dr. John Yiamouyiannis, titled "**Fluoride, The Aging Factor".** He documents how fluoride alters the body's production of collagen, which is the connective tissue between the cells and our joints, as well as affecting our arteries and our skin.

Remember all that plaque buildup inside our arteries? Well, it can only build up if the arteries are not smooth and are partially damaged.

He also points out that **fluoride can cause autoimmune disease** and alternations in our DNA repair mechanisms, which make up the building blocks of our genes and cells. Did you ever wonder how cells start mutating, leading to uncontrolled growth and cancer? There has to be a trigger or multiple triggers.

Just think about it. **Would you have thought forty years ago that people would be making money selling water**? At first it was the high end, fancy-smancy European waters that were drunk for their mineral content. Then later you started seeing water machines in supermarkets. Now, there is bottled water everywhere. Most in plastic bottles.

Why are people buying bottled water when they can be drinking it free out of the tap? Why? Because the mass population is much smarter than you think. They realize that you have to start with something pure, especially if it is a solvent to all the other foods you eat and causes you to absorb everything and filter out all the waste through your kidneys.

These **contaminants** are really scary. We thought we would do a good job in cleaning up our air by putting catalytic converters on our cars and changing the gasoline to make it lead-free and so forth. Well, they put an additive into our gasoline called MTBE, which is so darn toxic that it infiltrates the ground water and has been found in varying amounts in all fifty states.

A European study linked MTBE to liver and kidney tumors in mice. While we have clean burning gasoline with this stuff, we're being poisoned internally. You figure it out. Maybe that's why everyone is buying bottled water.

I'll go one step further, distilled water. **Distilled water combined with a charcoal filter removes just about all the impurities**. You are left with a perfect solvent for dissolving your organic minerals and nutrients, bathing yourself internally with clean, pure water that will not change its chemical consistency or produce mutations due to its toxic load. Many of my arthritis patients drink distilled water to help alleviate the arthritic symptoms. You see, it all starts with water.

Most of us assume that the food and water we drink is safe for consumption. After all we have the FDA in the USA to look out for us right? Think again. In 2015 a series of articles came out about Marines that lived at the marine base in Camp Lejeune North Carolina. Researchers noticed that they had a higher than normal rate of male breast cancer which is very rare. Breast Cancer is something that is usually associated with women not men. As research continued into the matter there was growing suspicion that the water supply had been contaminated with very small quantities of discarded petroleum products. So, how safe is our water?

During my travels, I ran into a fellow RVer traveling solo in a Class B motorhome like mine. When I interviewed this lady, I found out that she was an independent thinker from northern California willing to stick her neck out and explore the world. When our conversation got to doctors, she rarely uses them. The last time she went she was told that she had hypothyroidism and would need to take thyroid hormone. She did research on it and started drinking distilled water and eating a lot of fruits and vegetables and no processed food. Guess what? She told me that when she returned to the doctor to get re tested, her thyroid had returned to normal.

Some of you may be saying, "I heard distilled water is bad for you because it doesn't have any minerals." Let me answer that.

The minerals that you absorb are organic minerals. That means they have been absorbed in their organic shape from the ground through vegetables and fruits and transformed into a food that we can use biologically. We don't have the same mechanisms as plants to transform inorganic minerals to organic minerals. We may have a little bit of an ability to do that, but it's minimal compared to the benefits we get from eating organic minerals through vegetables and fruits. Maybe that's why some of those vitamin-mineral studies came back negative because they contained nonbioavailable inorganic minerals?

If you can't afford a distiller for your house, then maybe a **reverse osmosis system** is the next best thing. It has a very high filtration rate through the micro pore membranes through which the water is squeezed. There are other forms of cartridge filters around, which are good; however, the distillation process and the reverse osmosis system are probably the best.

Did you know that distilled water even enhances your mineral absorption rate? Distilled water will not conduct electricity when two parts inorganic minerals or less are present. The reason distilled water is used in car batteries is to keep the lead plates from breaking down as fast.

Just think about it, distilled water has two parts inorganic minerals or less, while the average American tap water ranges between 350 to 1000 parts per million of contaminants. Remember that one part per million created six-hundred-quadrillion toxic molecules. I think you are starting to get the picture.

The purer the water, the less contamination you get into your body.

I have always found it interesting how they measure the safety of toxins, for example, aluminum, arsenic, chloride, cobalt, lead, or even nitrates. They generally feed this stuff to animals and find out at what level 50% of them die. Pretty scientific, huh?

Well, they can't feed it to humans so they have to give it to rats or mice or guinea pigs or something like that. Then, they come out with a statement "... This chemical is safe at so many parts per million." Okay, I'll buy that.

Then they do another study with another chemical that they decide to add, such as, let's say, aspartame, or anything like that, and they say, "Okay we can take so much of that and it doesn't cause any problems right now. Of course, we don't know if it will cause any problems five generations down the line, but right now, it doesn't cause any problems." Have they heard of the science of Epigenetics? What we do in our reproductive years, influences the health of several generations down line.

They take another chemical, do the same thing, and eventually if you read the label on a jar of stuff you buy, it has thirty different chemicals in it. You buy another product, which has twenty different chemicals. You eat in a restaurant where they use normal tap water run through lead pipes or whatever and that has a whole slew of its own chemicals. Then you go outside and breathe the exhaust of the cars whizzing by, and that have another whole set of polluting chemicals, which your lungs absorb, you know the stuff they call smog.

Then you go into your office building and it has what is known as Sick Building Syndrome. On your way home from the office, the lawn has just been sprayed with some kind of organophosphate fertilizer or maybe even a pesticide, and you get a whiff of that. By the time you get home, **you may have accumulated a hefty dose of chemicals which have been deemed "safe" individually, but in combination and cumulatively, they may play major havoc on your immune system and your ability to age healthy**.

You see, the chronic chemical exposure from all the toxins that are out there, which our body is not designed to detoxify because the toxins did not exist while we were evolving, is **causing a gradual stress on your system**. This toxic stress reaches a point where the cells just cannot handle it anymore, and you start getting sick, very, very sick.

Is that the way you want to live? In this toxic environment? **Living with toxic water does not lead to healthy aging. Get out of that pollution, and start drinking pure healthy water**. You can use a distiller, a reverse osmosis filter or get high quality filtered bottled water.

I was reading a recent article from the Associated Press, entitled "**Lymphoma Rising Baffling**, But New Therapies in Sight". It stated that this mysterious immune system cancer has been making a quiet comeback and rates have nearly doubled since the seventies. It questioned if diet was to blame, pesticides, air pollution, viruses, obesity . . . Nobody knows, so the article says, and they are launching major studies to discover what's behind the rapid rise of this type of cancer.

Well, **it is a cancer of the immune system** and obviously we are taking something internally that is decreasing our resistance. Another way of looking at it is that we are not taking enough of the right nutrients internally to increase our resistance. Just as I stated before, "Garbage in, garbage out."

People are fortifying their immune systems with paper houses. Any wind that comes along will blow that house over. **More and more people are becoming aware of the dangers of pesticides, chemicals, heavy metal toxicity, GMO's (genetic engineered foods), and are demanding organically grown foods.**

As a matter of fact, the U.S. Federal Government is attempting to define and regulate organic foods, by defining **"organic" as something that does not have genetically modified ingredients, is not irradiated to decontaminate the product, and sewage sludge has not been utilized as fertilizer**. This is just a minor start in an avalanche of future discovery that the food we consume is slowly poisoning us. Why did it take so long for artery-clogging trans fats to be banned from our food chain? If you see a label saying partially hydrogenated fats, they are trans fats.

Walter Willett, chairman of the department of nutrition at Harvard University's school of public health stated, "This was really the biggest food processing disaster ever. The human toll has got to be in the millions."

Partially hydrogenated oils have been used since the 1940's because they made food last longer. They were thought to be actually safer than natural saturated fats such as butter. Ever wonder why pastries would last forever? Why do processed foods such as packaged cookies, crackers, cakes, soft buns, pizza dough, vegetable shortening, hard margarine, pre mixes such as frostings, pancake mix, chocolate mix, French fries, tortilla, corn and potato chips, chicken nuggets, snack foods, microwave popcorn and soft breads last a long time? Its trans fats.

The food industry loved trans fats. They increased the shelf life of food and made the food cheaper to produce. Fast food chains only recently banned trans fats from their products. How long have we been eating these artery clogging products? The agribusiness food industry slowly introduces chemicals into your body. These chemicals gradually clogs up your body with chemicals and byproducts from those chemicals. At a well-known pediatric research hospital's Grand Rounds, I asked the lecturer, "Why is autism growing in our population". He answered, "Environmental toxins".

It took a lawsuit in 2015 from a 100 year old scientist Dr. Fred Kummerow, a University of Illinois professor to finally get the FDA to put a ban on these products. He has been researching trans fats for 60 years and warning about their dangers in clogging arteries. He was able to develop arterial sclerosis in rats by giving them trans fats. When the trans fats were removed from the rats diet, the arteriosclerosis went away.

This is an excellent example of the friendly foods that we have been eating may slowly be killing us. I noticed this at the northern Canadian Newfoundland Labrador border with the **epidemic of childhood obesity.**

Talking to knowledgeable people in the area, community nurses, doctors, social workers, the problem **started occurring when the children started eating western fast foods**. Computers, computer games, lack of exercise and the sedentary lifestyle also contributed to this childhood obesity epidemic. It was rare for me to see a thin teenager in that region. You would think an area that's specializes in fishing would have healthy people, that was not what I found. The social worker at a long term care home told me that she is seeing younger and younger people coming into her facility.

Where was our government all these years while we've been slowly poisoned by this processed artificially enhanced food we've been eating? Just follow the money.

The major food companies aren't standing still either. They see money to be made in natural foods and they're all jumping into the arena. For example, Nestle USA joined the natural and functional food niche with the introduction of dietary supplements. H. J. Heinz Company also formed an organic and nutritional food unit. Quaker Oats, another large company, got involved in the functional food business, which is designed to offer specific health benefits above basic nutrition.

Did you know that General Mills, Inc., Kraft Foods, Inc., and Kellogg's Company have all gotten into this wellness arena, and they have been gobbling up smaller companies that have been in the health food industry?

We have companies specializing in unprocessed organic foods springing up all over the place. Even the major grocery chains have organic sections.

What's happening is as the consumer becomes savvy about pesticides and genetically modified foods, the baby-boomers want to live longer and they're searching out the health benefits of foods.

Baby boomers want to stay healthy and active into old age and they know that food has something to do with the disease processes we are all experiencing. The big companies, sensing a market, are all getting into it.

Sales within the organic and natural food industry have grown fifteen to twenty percent per year, compared to one to two percent for general grocery merchandising. In Europe, where they have the massive protests against genetically engineered foods (GMO's), sales of natural foods are growing even faster. Europeans have always been health-oriented and they're rebelling against artificial ingredients, preferring pure, unadulterated sources as building blocks for cells.

All this change in the food industry is good for you, the consumer. It is going to create greater competition and a larger selection of healthy foods that you can buy. Since the government is going to be regulating it to a certain extent, hopefully they will have more and more rules in the future, but it is a good start in the right direction.

Maybe someday you will be able to get a choice of supplements, probiotics or digestive enzymes as your after dinner treat at a fancy restaurant instead of the traditional mint to help you digest your food. They may still be mint-flavored, however, they'll be designed to augment nutritionally the food you just consumed so that you will have balanced nutrition at every meal. Is this Utopia or is this a possibility?

Talking about utopia, the first time I re-wrote this chapter was on spectacular Marble Mountain in southern Cape Breton Island, Nova Scotia Canada. There is an overlook rest stop high above the absolutely gorgeous Bras d' Or Lake, a UNESCO biosphere Reserve. When I say spectacular, I mean spectacular with fluffy clouds, distant islands and breathtaking views. The closest places in the USA with similar views that I have been to, are Crater Lake Oregon, and Lake Tahoe at the Nevada – California border.

When I was in Sopot, Poland, recently, the doctor at the local clinic after prescribing antibiotics, also prescribed vitamins and healthy probiotic bacteria to replenish the ones destroyed by the antibiotic. Now that's progressive integrative medicine.

Let's get back down to earth and discuss what you can do food-wise to get the best nutrients possible in the foods you eat. While you have always heard the saying that you should be eating at least five servings of fruits and vegetables per day to be divided by three servings of vegetables and two servings of fruit or more a day, how do you choose?

I like to think of it as **a beautiful rainbow** going over the water, and there is a pot of gold at the end of that rainbow. But, the trick is, you have to eat the rainbow to reach the pot of gold. **Just as bees and various insects are attracted to colors in fruit for pollination, we should be attracted to colors in vegetables and fruits for sustentation.** Generally the brighter the color of something, the more vitamins and minerals it has to enhance our health. The duller the food, the less nutrients it has.

So what are the colors of the rainbow? Red, orange, yellow, green, blue, indigo, violet—beautiful colors. What foods can you think of that follow that rainbow scheme?

Let's start with **red**. Think hard, what is red. I know it's on the tip of your tongue. How about tomatoes, cherries, strawberries, cranberries, pomegranate.

Did you know that strawberries and tomatoes are high in vitamin C. Cherries are high in bioflavonoids, as are other berries? Cherries also contain rutin.

Tomatoes contain melatonin and licopene which is one of the seven hundred carotenoids present in fruits and vegetables. **Licopene** may be protective against prostate cancer, as well as being a potent antioxidant. Strawberries also contain licopene, a cancer-fighter.

Orange. Well, the most common thing we think of is an orange, a citric acid fruit that is very high in vitamin C, protective to the immune system. How about carrots and yams, which contain vitamin A and beta-carotene. Carrots are important for maintaining your eye sight.

Yellow. There are a number of vegetables that are yellow. Squash and beans are high in **choline**, essential in building the neurotransmitters (acetyl choline) that help keep our nervous system in tune, along with the B vitamins. How about bananas. Did you know bananas contain melatonin, which boosts our immune system and helps us sleep better? Onions contain selenium, which works together with the potent antioxidant, vitamin E.

Green. That's a big one. **Green is the color of nature**. It is the color of chlorophyll, the substance in green vegetables and plants and trees, which transforms sunlight into energy. I bet you never thought of that. Without chlorophyll and without the sunlight, we would not be able to live. The green fruits and vegetables are extremely important to us. Cruciferous vegetables, such as cabbage, kale, brussel sprouts, broccoli, even may have anticancer effects. Broccoli, which you have heard a lot about, contains chromium, which helps maintain our insulin levels. Avocados contain magnesium, which is helpful in protecting the heart and boosting our memory.

Dark green leafy vegetables are very high in carotene. Beta-carotene has potent antioxidant properties. Dark green vegetables also contain a lot of vitamin E, as well as vitamin K, which is essential for normal blood clotting.

How about rutin, which is found in green peppers, as well as under the skins of citrus fruits. It is a bioflavonoid, which may be essential in suppressing tumors of the colon and helps fight increased cholesterol. It even helps in the absorption of vitamin C.

There are too many health benefits from all the greens to mention in this book, but some of the important greens are cucumbers, collard greens, brussel sprouts, broccoli, cabbage (cabbage has been used as an anti-cancer and diet food), lettuces, spinach, turnip greens and collards.

Blue. There are a number of fruits and even vegetables that have a blue color from blueberries to squashes. **Blueberries** are very potent anti-oxidants and are **considered a super food**. How about the purple cabbage, which is loaded with nutrients. Blue-green algae is a popular supplement for detoxification programs. It is a potent antioxidant and anti-inflammatory agent.

As you can see from the examples given, the colors are important. Not only do they have medicinal and preventative health properties, they are also essential sources of organic minerals, as well as vitamins, along with enzymes such as **papain**, which is in **papaya**, which aids in digestion.

Papain is **essential in the digestion of proteins** and has been prescribed in Germany for years to aid in digestion and heartburn after big meals.

Did you know that papaya and pineapple also contain **bromelain**, which reduces inflammation and enhances immune function, fighting allergies and other inflammatory immune diseases?

Bromelain is essential in the digestion of starches and has been used as an **anti-inflammatory agent**. It is thought to reduce chronic inflammation, such as in arthritis and blood vessels, which can lead to fatty deposits. So, maybe you should eat papaya and pineapple whenever you get a chance?

The **rainbow foods**, as I call them, are a good way for you to pick fruits and vegetables. Salmon, an excellent protein source high in Omega-3 fatty acids (which fight arteriosclerosis), is also red.

When you go shopping, just remember, **the brighter the color, the better it is for you.**

Eat fresh colors and you will be healthy, but make sure this stuff is not sprayed, and wash it thoroughly when you get home. You don't know what they've put on it to maintain its color. Sometimes they spray or gas these vegetables and fruits to maintain their color so they'll have a longer shelf life. Just one more trick the food industry uses that may destroy the nutritional benefits of what we eat. (I've heard some horror stories of what grocers used to do years ago to keep old ground beef looking red.)

Let's get into more specific anti-aging foods. It is impossible in this book to cover the nutritional value of every single food. If you are interested, I recommend you go to the library and get some books on nutrition, primarily from the dietetic point of view, and they will break down every single food and every single vitamin that it contains. You can also use the USDA or NIH web sites for information.

There is a lot of confusion on the internet with snippets of data being thrown at you from all sides. It is best to look at published textbooks or research articles in well-known journals written by PhD's or MD's and other doctors that specialize in nutrition. Unless an article is peer reviewed, it does not stand the scrutiny of science. Anyone can say anything, if it is repeated enough it becomes established truth without proof. Remember that researcher I went to see? His research was referenced all over but when I went to see the proof, the data, Poof it had vanished and the article was retracted by the journal.

In the next section of this chapter, I will cover specific foods, which I believe are beneficial in longevity and give you the rationale behind them.

This afternoon as I was dictating the first edition of this chapter on a porch filled with radiant warm Florida sunshine, I snacked occasionally on a pear, banana, or apple, which kept my sugar at a constant level, also filling me with essential vitamins. For supper, which I just finished, I had the rainbow foods.

I had a delicious carrot salad mixed with oranges from our back yard for flavor, along with a little cinnamon. It was absolutely delicious and it gave me a tremendous amount of vitamins. I also had artichoke leaves and hearts, which gave me the greens. For protein and grains, I had spaghetti with the meatballs having multigrain bread fortified with bran in them. As you can see from this meat, I am not a vegetarian and occasionally eat red meat but mostly stick to chicken and fish. However, my diet consists primarily of large quantities of fruits, vegetables and salads.

For protein I use various beans, lentils, primarily skinless chicken breasts, fish, of which I recommend salmon and other cold water fish the most. Sardines and herring have higher concentrations of omega 3 and 6 fatty acids in them. I limit my consumption of lean beef.

I also make tofu shakes, veggie burgers, and quite a few fruit shakes made in my high-powered blender. **I prefer whole food shakes compared to extracted juices because of the roughage and the added nutrients from the skins of fruits and vegetables. Whole fruit shakes produce slower balanced absorption of the fructose**. Many fruits have most of the vitamins in the skins. The problem with juices is the high concentration of fructose sugar that gets into your bloodstream real fast. You do not want to have a high fructose load all at once. The excess sugar turns into fat. Because of rapid fructose absorption and high concentrations of corn syrup in everything we eat and drink, people get fat.

It is much better to eat the entire fruit so the fructose sugars are metabolized slowly. When a diabetic has a hypoglycemic effect due low blood sugar, a glass of orange juice will perk them right up. The fructose sugar in orange juice gets absorbed immediately. Whole fruit sugars take longer for absorption and don't get into our cells as fast. On the world cruise I saw a man at the table in front of me go into a hypoglycemic seizure with a full glass of orange juice sitting in front of him. I helped immediately. He didn't drink his orange juice on time to prevent the seizure.

While I am on this topic, I do want to mention **that steaming is far preferable to boiling anything, because when you boil something you lose most of the minerals through the boiled water**. Lightly steaming vegetables preserves most of the nutrients. You can also use the waterless cookware that slowly cooks the vegetables with almost no water, maintaining all its nutrients. I do not recommend canned vegetables and fruits except in emergencies, because most of the nutrients are blanched out. However, canned tomatoes do retain many nutrients.

One of my active retired patients taught me how to get the most vitamins out of vegetables as easily as possible: Buy flash frozen multi-vegetables that you can microwave or steam lightly and have just about all the nutrients that are in fresh vegetables. Since he is single, it is an easy way for him to get a large variety of all his vegetables fairly rapidly and the blended variety makes it taste very good.

Through his ingenuity, he found a practical, useful solution to keep himself healthy. **By the way, he is eighty years old, walks over a thousand miles a year and dances a couple of times a week, a clever man.**

Bran

I feel bran is an important aspect of the longevity program because **it keeps things moving in your gut**. It is a great source of roughage and, believe it or not, **it is non-caloric fiber containing vitamins, such as riboflavin, thiamin, pantothenic acid, B1, B6, and niacin.**

Bran is not the grain itself, but the coating of the seeds of grain, the shells of the seeds, such as oats or wheat. It has been proven to relieve constipation, prevent diverticulitis, and has been known to stabilize cholesterol levels and decrease blood sugars for diabetics. But, the thing I like most about it is its propulsive effects. Food has to pass through your system and not hang around too much. If it hangs around a great deal, it promotes putrification and causes all kinds of intestinal problems, which can lead to colon cancer. **By maintaining regular bowel movements with good consistency and decreasing your blood sugar and cholesterol levels, you are getting a healthy aging nutritional effect.**

While we are on that subject, don't forget to **get your colonoscopy**. A doctor friend of mine had to talk me into having mine done. I had mine without anesthesia, slight discomfort, but I enjoyed watching my own anatomy on the monitor and those "cool" microvilli that do all of the nutrient absorption. Colon Cancer is one of the most preventable cancers that we have. The polyps can be excised before they become cancerous.

Another grain that is beneficial is **oats or oatmeal**, which is also high in B vitamins, vitamin E, and various minerals, including iron. Additionally, oatmeal contains protein and very high concentrations of soluble fiber, which also assists in lowering your cholesterol.

So, here you have a couple of good foodstuffs you can have for breakfast oatmeal and bran muffins.

Cranberries

For your daily beverages, it is far better to have a mixture of a juice, such as cranberry juice and water, than any soft drinks or sugar drinks. I like cranberries as an anti-aging juice because it **helps prevent a problem quite common in the elderly, urinary tract infections**. If these things are not prevented, you can become very ill and develop a chronic septicemia, which can eventually lead to your death.

Cranberry juice seems to be effective against bladder and urinary tract infections, probably by inhibiting the growth of the bacteria in the uterine lining. Cranberry juice also helps lower blood pressure in animals.

One thing I like about it is that it really makes water, that I recommend drinking in large quantities, taste better. By protecting you from common infections of the urinary tract, you preserve your kidneys which filter the waste out of your system.

Garlic

I mentioned garlic previously for cold prevention along with ginseng, but I think it is so important as a longevity herb that I'll mention it again. Garlic needs to be a regular part of your anti-aging diet**. Not only is it antifungal, antibacterial, and antiviral, it may also protect you against liver damage, lower your serum cholesterol and triglyceride levels and your heart.** It has also been shown to **decrease platelet clotting, thereby thinning your blood** and reducing your risk of clot induced strokes. Have you ever wondered why the Mediterranean inhabitants have low cardiovascular diseases? One of the reasons is their high consumption of garlic and the other is consumption of extra virgin olive oil.

Did you know that along with onions and chives, garlic boosts immunity? It helps fight infections and prevents cancers. It also helps neutralize toxins and free radicals. Some people also use it as an anti-stress agent.

The medicinal use of garlic goes back as far as 6,000 years ago. It was used in Egypt and Rome, as well as in ancient Greece. **Hippocrates, the Greek Father of Medicine, recommended it as an antibiotic for infections**. It was also used during the plague in France as a preventative agent.

In 1858, Louis Pasteur, the famous French microbiologist, was able to kill bacteria grown in a dish with garlic juice and reported on it in the medical literature.

The stories about garlic go on and on and on. As unpleasant as it may taste to some people, I personally like to take it on a regular basis as part of my longevity program. My grandmother in Poland and my pharmacist aunt in Germany both used and recommended it for colds. My uncle used it for circulation and general health. Fresh, crushed, uncooked garlic being the best since crushing it releases enzymes. I like it on toast with tomatoes and oregano or chives for a pleasant sandwich. Aged garlic supplements is probably second best.

Soybeans

Soybeans are **probably the most versatile, beneficial product you can have for health preservation and life extension**.

Soy products, **a great substitute for animal protein**, should definitely be on your food list. You can buy it readily as protein powder or as a gelatinous substance known as tofu, which you can fry or mix with fruits, ice, and honey and make delicious shakes. The **isoflavones** in soy products lower the bad cholesterol (LDL), as well as triglycerides, and help raise the HDL portion of cholesterol, which is the good cholesterol.

The genistein portion of the isoflavones in soy has potent anti-cancer effects on laboratory animals. Besides that, the isoflavones in soybeans, which are glycetein, daidzein, and genistein, seem to work as **weak estrogens** in the body and are a great adjunct to any type of natural hormone replacement. Soybeans also contain phytates, which are active antioxidants and free radical scavengers.

In societies where diets are rich with soy products, there is a lowered incidence of cancer of all types. Soy is a complete protein, just as meat, and contains all the essential amino acids, making it an excellent meat protein substitute. We use it in our soy veggie burgers, which taste almost exactly like regular hamburgers. It's amazing.

You can also try **tempeh**, which is a soy product that is fermented and has the consistency of meat, making it an excellent additive for casseroles or other dishes in which you would use ground beef.

Regular soy milk is all right, but it is a taste you have to get used to. You can, however, purchase chocolate and vanilla flavored soy milk which is absolutely delicious, so go ahead and try it. I have also used almond milk on my cereal and in coffee.

With its many benefits from replacing estrogen levels in post-menopausal women to reducing cholesterol to its anti-cancer effects and being a perfect substitute for meat. You may consider soy as part of your longevity diet program. I recommend soy products routinely for my patients, especially those who are anemic and need higher protein intake to build up red blood cells, as well as muscles. My favorite soy products are Tofu mixed in a fruit shake and Soy Powders.

For women, the phytoestrogenetic activity of soy products may protect them against the risks of developing cancers due to high estrogen levels, such as breast cancer and uterine cancer, as well as benign breast cysts. You see, the **phytoestrogens from soy act like estrogens by occupying estrogen receptors and, therefore, they help regulate the estrogen level in a woman's body**, having a gentle, protective effect. In the Far East, women take as much as 100 mg to 200 mg of isoflavones a day. As we all know, they have a very, very low incidence of breast cancer compared to women in the United States. However, when they move to the United States and start adapting to our diet, the breast cancer rate increases dramatically. **Phytoestrogens are also found in nuts, seeds, whole grains, and beans.**

Genistein, a potent phytoestrogen found in soy, is also available in capsular form and is generally taken in quantities of 80 mg a day or less. However, I feel that the total soy product is more beneficial than just an isolated component.

As you can tell from my discussion of soy, there is not enough good I can say about it. It is such a valuable food source that it should be a component of your anti-aging food program. For what it's worth, a PhD good friend of mine who is a vegetarian, is often taken for being a 30 year old but he is actually 59 years old.

Oils

Our bodies need oils and essential fatty acids, but it is the type of oil we consume that is extremely important to how our body will metabolize it and use it as an energy source. Essential fatty acids, such as alpha-linolenic acid and gamma-linolenic acid, the highest concentration of which is found in **flax seed oil**, we absolutely need. Other sources are sesame seeds, walnuts, pumpkin seeds, and soybeans.

Returning to the rainbow colors for a moment, **dark green leafy vegetables also contain essential fatty acids**, however, not as high a concentration as **flax seed oil**. You can also get essential fatty acids in borage oil.

These products need to be refrigerated and they do have an oily smell to them. You may want to take them in a capsular form of up to 1,000 to 5,000 mg twice a day.

Why are these good fats so important? Because **they are essential fats and are totally opposite to bad**

fats. The transfats are found in high temperature cooking processes and the saturated fats are found in meat and dairy products.

Unsaturated fats are vegetable oils, which include soy oil, sunflower oil, olive oil, safflower oil, and oils found in grains, seeds, nuts, and legumes.

So, why take essential fatty acids? Well, essential fatty acids have been declining in our diet over the past seventy-five years and a lack of essential fatty acids in our diet can be a contributing factor to a large host of health problems ranging from inflammatory disorders to heart problems to arthritis. These essential fatty acids are nutrients, just like minerals and vitamins we take in and are important in maintaining life itself. The **Mediterranean diet** is considered one of the healthiest because it has unsaturated fats, extra virgin olive oil, along with fruits, vegetables, seeds and nuts.

To test the validity of the Mediterranean Diet, researchers in Spain devised a clever 6 year study which was known as the PREDIMED study. They pre-selected 7447 55-80 year old participants with cardiovascular risk factors such as obesity, diabetes, elevated blood pressure and so on. They had a known ad risk group of subjects to start with instead of random normal subject.

The cleverness of the study was that one group of participants was given a liter of virgin olive oil to use each week and another group was given mixed nuts of which they were told to eat an ounce per day. They were given foods to consume, instead of being told to just eat certain foods. The control group was told to eat a low fat diet with some other restrictions.

The reason that I am bring this study up was because the "Mediterranean diet" beat all expectations. The study was halted in 4.8 years because of remarkable results. They wanted the control group to benefit from those results. The researchers found that the extra virgin olive oil subjects had 30 percent reduction heart attack, stroke and cardiovascular disease than the low fat control group. The subjects that ate nuts, had 28 percent less incidents of stroke and heart attacks. Another benefit of this study was mental acuity. Cognition improved verses the low fat diet controls. It is hard to replicate those results with drugs. Just like Aristotle said "Let medicine be your food and let food be your medicine".

To follow up on the original results, a new Spanish multicenter PREDIMED-PLUS study was started comparing caloric restriction and physical activity subjects with the extra virgin olive oil and mixed nuts subjects.

The Mediterranean is rich in essential fatty acids. Essential fatty acids are used to manufacture cell membranes, which act as coverings for our cells and keep them from falling apart. **The stronger the covering, the more impenetrable it is to invading organisms**. The essential fatty acids are also important in the **manufacture of prostaglandins**, which act kind of like hormones in your body or like super enzymes and help regulate important functions, such as fertility, conception, blood pressure, heart rate, blood clotting, pressure and inflammation on eyes, joints and ears, affecting the immune system and the nervous system, such as thinking, mood, and automatic reactions, such as fight/flight mechanisms.

5001-LENH

They also affect the skin—moisture, healing properties, and secretions from various glands, as well as kidney functions, heart functions, temperature regulation, fat deposits, appetite, sensitivity to cold, and various tumors and the spread of tumors. In other words, **they affect every aspect of our body**.
That's why those essential fatty acids are essential.

Did you know that prostaglandins also regulate your inflammatory process and inflammation is important because if you have an infective agent, you need the inflammatory process to help ward off and fight that agent? The inflammatory reaction is a healing process. The prostaglandins kind of keep things in check and keep the inflammation from becoming too large and devouring your whole body.

Prostaglandins work in pairs. One set of prostaglandins, which comes basically from arachidonic acid, is an essential fatty acid available in most diets. The other part of the prostaglandins comes from the alpha-linoleic acid and the gamma-linoleic acid, which are in short supply in our diet. Together they suppress the inflammatory response, keeping the inflammation in check. If you don't have enough of the essential fatty acids, which come from flax seed oils and other sources mentioned previously, and which regulates the inflammatory response, you may have an inflammation that goes out of control, such as allergic reactions and so forth.

As you can see, **the essential fatty acids are a very important component of your immune system and help trigger a variety of important functions in your body, such as clot formation, allergic reactions, stimulate hormone production, as well as control smooth muscles and tissues swelling.**

Did you know they use prostaglandins to induce labor in childbirth? That's how important these hormone-like substances are, and **they are derived from these essential fatty acids**, which you must have in your diet and should be an important component of your longevity program.

Studies have shown that women consuming high concentrations of essential fatty acids have lower cancer rates, including breast cancer.

Did you know that they even regulate stomach secretions? You need enough acid secretion in your stomach to digest your foods. If you don't digest food properly, you won't get all the nutrients from it. Sometimes an acidic food, such as a sour pickle or pickle juice, helps with the digestion. My 83 year old sister tells me to drink pickle juice after eating because it's good for digestion and sometimes indigestion if you ate too much food.

So, you can **get your essential fatty acids through a Mediterranean type diet or in the form of extra supplementation**. You can take them in capsules or you can take the oils and put them on salads. Either way is okay.

There are **two essential fatty acid families**, the **Omega-6** and the **Omega-3** fatty acids. For those of you really interested, the Omega-6 family includes linoleic acid, gamma-linolenic acid, and arachidonic acid. The Omega-3 family consists of alphalinolenic acid, eicosapentaenoic acid, and docosahexaenoic acid. All of these are essential fatty acids, which are broken down into the two families, with the Omega-3 family being especially cardio-protective.

Omega-3 fatty acids have gotten a lot of attention recently for being cardio-protective and studies have shown it to reduce LDL cholesterol, the bad cholesterol, as well as triglyceride levels. These Omega-3 fatty acids have also been shown to have antihypertensive effects on patients.

There have also been reports of people doing better with rheumatoid arthritis after taking Omega-3 fatty acids. Sources of Omega-3 fatty acids include linseed oil and evening primrose oil, as well as flax seed oil which contains the essential fatty acids. One of the most common sources are **fish oils** from oily fish, such as **salmon, cod, mackerel, herring, and sardines**. I give my patients neutral-tasting cod liver oil, which has a slight lemon flavor and contains very high concentrations of eicosapentaenoic acid and docosahexaenoic acid, as a protection for their cardiovascular systems.

There is a debate about consuming large quantities of fish to get your Omega-3 fatty acids because fish are constantly exposed to toxins, especially in coastal areas. Therefore, you need to **stick to cold water fish species, such as salmon, tuna, cod, mackerel, and haddock, as well as herring**, and avoid fish from industrialized or polluted coastal waters, which may have high concentrations of contaminants. Besides, you can get your Omega-3 fatty acids from the flax seed oil and soy oil, as well as from vegetables and beans.

If you think you are getting protection by ordering a deep fried fish burger in a fast food store, think again. The **deep-frying of the fish destroys the Omega-3 fatty acids and the high temperature of the grease causes trans fatty acids, which clog up arteries with free radicals, which increase your aging process**. Do yourself a big favor: Stick to the cold water fish, such as salmon, or take a good-tasting cod liver oil.

Omega-3 fatty acid products, as well as essential fatty acid products, can be found at your local health food store. However, if you get cod liver oil, taste is always a problem. Make sure you get an oil that tastes neutral or has no flavor whatsoever, **because if it doesn't taste good, you aren't going to take it**. It took me a long time to find a product that actually tasted good and that patients would take without complaining.

Let's review the type of oils you should avoid and the type of oils you should take.

Avoid saturated fats, which is the stuff that makes meat taste good. It's the stuff that burns on the barbecue grill. It's the drippings from sausage, bacon, and chicken skins.

When eating animal proteins, avoid the fats and get as lean a portion as possible.

Absolutely do not deep-fry anything. You need the oils, but you need them from the right sources.

One interesting finding of the PREDIMED study was that even though the Mediterranean diet was rich in fats, 48% of energy used, the participants did not gain weight nor abdominal fat. This shows the importance of using the right kinds of oils. People are getting fat from high fructose corn syrup and carbohydrates in their diet, not from fats. The Adkins diet high in fats and proteins, but low in carbohydrates causes weight loss.

You want to have unsaturated oils, which come from vegetable sources. You also need essential fatty acids, which come from flax seed oil and other oils. **For cardiac protection, stick to the Omega-3 fatty acid foods**.

The **best source of vegetable protein is soy protein**, which also contains isoflavones and has a myriad of beneficial health effects.

So, **what exactly is the Mediterranean diet** that is giving us all those cardiovascular protective results? 1. Use lots of olive oil for cooking, on salads, baking etc. 2. High consumption of fruits, legumes, vegetables, mixed nuts and cereals. 3. Moderate intake of wine, especially red wine, with the main meal. Since there is a debate as to how much wine is safe, maybe one glass? 4. Moderate consumption of fish, seafood, fermented dairy products (for the probiotics), such as yogurt, Kefir, which is fermented milk and cheese. 5. Poultry and eggs. 6. Low intake of red and processed meats and sweets.

Ancel Keys, the University of Minnesota physiologist and inventor of the World War 2 K-rations, ate a Mediterranean diet. When he retired, he moved to southwest Italy where people walked a lot and ate foods they grew. Keys died just shy of his 101st birthday and his wife died at 97. Keys was the originator of the diet-heart hypothesis where LDL cholesterol and saturated fats were the bad actors in Metabolic Syndrome. Statin cholesterol lowering medications are being written like candy by traditionally trained internists. However, cardiovascular disease remains the number one cause of death in developed countries.

Over 20 newer studies are starting to question this entire hypothesis. They are discovering that the real culprit is sugar. It was easy to blame butter, eggs, cheese and milk for cardiovascular disease since they were not the real big money makers for corporations. Sugar in its various forms is the goose that laid the golden egg. Prior to 1900 Cardiovascular Disease was rare and so was nonalcoholic fatty liver disease and diabetes. Since then the Metabolic Syndrome diseases have become the number one health problem in developed countries. Butter, cheese and milk have been staples of people's diets for thousands of years without major cardiovascular complications but sugar has not. Since the advent of sucrose and high fructose based foods, cardiovascular disease, stroke, dementia, obesity and diabetes have skyrocketed. Newer clinical trials on saturated fats, available on the NIH website, are showing that saturated fats are not the real culprit in heart disease, sugar is. The 10% dietary cap on saturated fats is not supported by the newer evidence. What a shocker, since 1950 we have been told to stop eating butter and eat margarine instead. Just follow the money.

Grains, Breads, and Starches

Just like good cholesterol and bad cholesterol, **there are good grains and bad grains.**

What are the **bad grains**? Anything bleached and highly processed, such as white bread or white rice.

What are the **good grains**? Anything that is whole and left alone as it is in nature and contains large quantities of fiber and complex carbohydrates, as well as vitamins and minerals.

Did you know that **whole rye bread contains more minerals, vitamins, and protein than whole wheat bread**? I remember growing up as a child in Europe where we ate whole rye bread. It was totally different than the mushy stuff you buy in the grocery store today. What we are buying is processed rye bread. Read the ingredients if it is all rye or wheat with some rye.

Whole rye bread has much more protein, phosphorous, calcium, iron, thiamin, niacin, and other vitamins and minerals than processed rye bread. As mentioned previously, it is more nutritious than whole wheat bread.

Try to get the whole rye kernel rather than the processed rye kernel, and the taste will be amazing.

Rice is a common food used throughout the world. Did you know that **one pound of white rice contains four times the food energy as the same weight of potatoes**? The problem with white rice is that the husk, bran, and germ are removed, leaving a product that is mostly starch.

The **best form of rice is brown rice**, which also contains the bran and the germ component of it, which is rich in B vitamins and iron.

Wheat is probably the most common grain used in the United States. The problem with it, again, is that it has been refined and people have become allergic to it due to its high prevalence.

Therefore, **it is good to alter the grains in your diet.**

Corn is a potent nutrient in our diet and is grown extensively throughout the world. It contains complex carbohydrates and essential vitamins, such as riboflavin and niacin, however, it **lacks two essential amino acids, lysine and tryptophan**, **which have to be supplemented from other sources**. Basically, pure corn on the cob is a good form of carbohydrate starch. Did you know that **corn on the cob is a low calorie food?**

High Fructose Corn syrup is used as a sweetener in many processed foods and soft drinks. If you read the labels **almost everything has corn syrup as a sweetener in it**. Ever wonder why there is such a high incidence of diabetes and now even juvenile diabetes in young children? **Carbohydrates lead to obesity and sugar leads to obesity.** We consume way too much of both willingly or unwillingly through Fructose and Corn syrup adulterated foods. That's why we have an obesity pandemic.

Potatoes are an excellent low-calorie source of food. They are loaded with carbohydrates and, if you **eat the skin, you will get a large dose of vitamins, as well as protein**. In Europe, the potato is a mainstay of essential minerals and vitamins.

I remember hearing stories that during World War II, the prisoners in the gulags of Russia were given potato peels, while the guards ate the potatoes. The prisoners were eating a healthier meal than the guards, allowing them to survive the cold bitter winters of Siberia and make it home after the war.

The only thing you have to remember about potatoes, to get all the nutrition you need, keep the skin on and don't add fat. Eat potatoes in moderation since they are high in carbohydrates.

A good example of a protective food is naturally fermented cabbage.

In 2005 researchers in Poland discovered that Polish Female immigrants to the USA were experiencing a breast cancer rate three times higher than those living in Poland. They knew that the cause had to be environmental. After careful observation of the polish women living in Detroit and Chicago, they notice that in Poland the women were consuming 30 pounds of naturally lacto fermented sauerkraut per year while in the USA they only ate 10 lbs. The natural fermentation process increases the bioavailability of nutrients in the cabbage which act as a protective mechanism against breast cancer.

Sauerkraut contains high levels of **glucosinolates** which have been found to have **anti-cancer properties** in the laboratory and apparently in humans, as observed in the polish women immigrant research. Glucosinolates may protect against DNA damage and restrict cancer cell growth. Research is being conducted at the University of New Mexico to determine how that process works. Dorothy Rybaczyk-Pathak from the University of New Mexico and Scientists at Michigan State University and the National Food and Nutrition Institute of Warsaw, Poland, concluded that "Women who ate at least three servings a week of raw- or short-cooked cabbage and sauerkraut had a significantly reduced breast cancer risk compared with those who only ate one serving per week"

It is important that the sauerkraut be naturally fermented and not artificially through chemicals. You can find natural sauerkraut in the refrigerated sections of your grocery store.

Another food with similar gut health qualities is Kimchi, the Korean version of sauerkraut. Kimchi is a naturally fermented blend of vegetables usually containing cabbage, salt, garlic, onions, red peppers, ginger, celery, carrots or other vegetables.

Cabbage and sauerkraut help to restore our gut flora that is often decimated by antibiotics.

The newest buzzword in biochemical research is our "**human microbiome**". The human microbiome is a diverse world of microorganisms that inhabit our bodies and promote our health. The US National Institute of Health is just now starting to study which microorganisms are associated with healthy humans and which with unhealthy humans. The larger the diversity of our gut flora, all working together through checks and balances, the healthier we humans may be.

It turns out that our gut environment, as shown through the sauerkraut observations, is far more important than regular doctors ever thought. If they knew how important our gut flora was for health, they would not have prescribe antibiotics for every sniffle that patients came in for. Antibiotics not only kill the bad bacteria but also the good bacteria in our gut that keep us healthy. Restoring a diverse gut flora through fermented foods and probiotics is extremely important for our overall health.

Fermented Sauerkraut, Kimchi, various yogurt strains, sour milk and other probiotic strains will go a long way towards restoring your gut flora to a healthier environment.

A PhD friend of mine had a visiting professor from the Czech Republic in Europe go to a doctor in the USA for a bad flu. After the doctor gave her a prescription for antibiotics he sent her on her way. The professor asked what are you going to give me as a probiotic? The US doctor stood dumbfounded, she explained that in Europe when a doctor gives you an antibiotic he will also give you a probiotic to restore your natural gut flora. You take the antibiotic first for 10 days and then take the probiotic so that you have biodiversity in your gut and the bad bacteria, such as clostridium difficile (C. Diff.), doesn't overgrow your gut and kill you.

This overgrowth happened to a cousin of mine after elective cardiac surgery in Jacksonville, Florida. He was discharged from the hospital and in three days readmitted because of declining health. By the time they figured out what was wrong, clostridium difficile, C. Diff., had overgrown his entire gut and bloodstream killing him in a few days. The prophylactic antibiotics he had before surgery had killed his good gut bacteria that balanced the C. Diff. The antibiotics did not kill all the C. Diff. After surgery the C. Diff multiplied unopposed by other organisms in the gut overloading his system and rapidly killing him.

There is a good reason why the USA is ranked 37h in overall health out of 181 countries by the WHO (World Health Organization), even though we spend the highest percentage of our GDP on our health care compared to other countries. In 2020 the US spent 18.8% and in 2022 17.3%. Out of high income countries, the USA was last. Maybe the other countries are practicing better preventive medicine and not just focusing on high ticket items that pay the most? France provides the overall best health care followed by Italy, Spain, Oman, Australia and Japan. Maybe the USA is developing into a health business country rather than a health care country?

Since my first book 20 years ago, a great deal of interest on gut bacterial flora composition (microbiome or biome) has developed in the microbiological science world. Older estimates of the number of distinct gut organisms were in the 500 range. This number came through growing bacteria in petri dishes that only showed the most common organisms. Newer studies at Stanford University done by the David Relman group, used pyrosequencing through DNA tags. Their research increased that distinct organism number in your gut to 5,600. That's a lot of different organisms consisting of about 100 trillion gut microbes. They all work together as a symphony eating up our digested food, producing vitamins, fine tuning our immune system and keeping the bad bacteria in check. Studies also show that as gut bacteria diversity increases, anxiety and depression decreases. Social ability and personality are also affected by gut bacteria diversity.

It appears that at least two of the bacteria in your gut produce a neurotransmitter called GABA. Behavioral conditions such as mood, neuroticism and autism have been correlated with the composition of the gut bacteria microbiome. The type of bacteria in your gut may make a difference in how you feel. The vagus nerve runs directly from your brain to your gut and can theoretically relay messages from your gut bacteria to your brain. These messages could be a crosstalk network signaling your brain to form certain chemicals that influence a host of physiological function in your body from how you feel to the metabolism of your food and nutrient absorption.

There is an epiphany going on in endocrinology right now. Endocrinology used to be associated with the secretory organs that produced all kinds of hormones, such as testosterone, estrogen, growth hormone and so on. Now, it appears that almost all cells in the body talk to one another, including all those little bugs that live in your gut, how interesting! Not to get too carried away, your gut microbiome is extremely important to your overall health in healthy aging. So, make sure that you have a diverse blend of bacteria living inside you, cheering you on to live longer.

For the newest updates on gut microflora research and how to replenish your gut bacteria biodiversity, refer to immunological and gastrological journals. You can also just search on line for **microbiome research**. The field of immunology is changing rapidly and the microbiome is a big part of it.

What should you eat? The US government department of health, (www.health.gov/dietary guidelines), officially released their new guidelines. These guidelines took a reverse course from previous guidelines. Now it is OK to have cholesterol from eggs. Saturated fats found in fatty meats and high fat dairy products increase blood cholesterol more than dietary cholesterol in eggs do.

The **sugars are the culprit**. No more than 10 percent of your calories should be from sugars. Sugars are in all processed foods, sauces, relishes, ketchup and dressing we eat. One can of soda will max out your sugar limit of 50 grams/day. If you add breads and cookies to that, you are way over the limit and the pounds start piling up around your hips, your belly and abdominal fat.

I know a lady that was thin her whole life until after retiring when she took up baking breads and cookies. Guess what happened? 40 lbs. later she had to give all of her beautiful clothes away because "they shrunk". Carbohydrates will put on pounds; increase your blood sugar and blood pressure faster than a speeding bullet.

The solution is simple. Do not keep carbohydrate foods in the house. That means pastries, cookies, donuts, white bread, crackers and snack foods. You can have high density multigrain bread in your freezer with which you make toast each day, but eating lots of bread piles on the carbs which piles on the fat just like sugars pile on the fat. Whole grains are good for you in cereals and don't forget to sprinkle flax seed on top of them for essential fatty acids.

Less meat, especially processed meat is beneficial for your cardiovascular health. Fish continue to be highly recommended for their omega 3,

6 fatty acids since they are cardio protective. **The cold water fatty fish along with sardines, herring and wild salmon** are loaded with those protective fatty acids.

How about salt? Most of us eat way too much salt. Salt stresses your cardiovascular system and can lead to high blood pressure. The new guidelines recommend no more than a teaspoon per day about 2300 milligrams, but for better heart protection stick to less than three quarter teaspoon, about 1500 milligrams. Read the labels for salt content and try to purchase less salty foods. You can also use a variety of spices for flavoring food rather than salt.

The guidelines also strongly emphasize 2.5 cups of mixed vegetables along with 2 cups of fruits. Just remember the rainbow colored foods that I talked about and you will do fine. Wine is good and the Mediterranean diet seems to be the healthiest. It's good to see that the new guidelines are more in line with what I talked about in 2000.

Juices

There are a large variety of juices used for longevity benefits and health promotion. The most common vitamin-rich juices we are familiar with are the citric juices with all the pulp, such as **grapefruit and orange**. I have mentioned previously the benefits of cranberry juice. People are even consuming aloe vera juice for its anti-inflammatory protective effects, both for your digestive system and applying it externally on sun burns. However, high fructose juices may be detrimental to your pre diabetic condition because of their high sugar load.

I have patients who attribute their strength and stamina in old age to **beet juice**. Others espouse benefits from cabbage juice.

You can make a juice from just about anything, from blueberries to cherries to limes to mulberries, to lemons, raspberries, prunes, pineapple, and watermelon. By the way, pure **watermelon juice** is very good tasting. It is an excellent thirst-quencher in the summer time and is loaded with vitamins.

Most of us drink orange juice, which has a high amount of fructose sugar, but there are many other juices and nectars available that taste fantastic and are healthy. The only problem is you have to **drink pure juice with pulp, not canned juice**, which contains high concentrations of corn syrup or fruit sweetener. The sweeteners are essentially sugar that is converted to fat in your body unless you burn it up as you're drinking it, through exercise.

If you are buying fruit juice, always buy pure fruit juice without any additives or sweeteners or anything labeled as a fruit drink. Try to avoid those flavored corn syrup drinks. Best of all, get the fruit and make your own fruit juice so you know what you're getting.

Pure fruit juices are a good way of getting lots of vitamins because they are so concentrated but carry a high sugar load. **Whole fruit juices** are even better because they also contain the skin and the pulp of the fruit which is a great source of roughage, as well as vitamins and minerals, which your body needs for your longevity program. The colored skin of the fruit or vegetable as previously mentioned, has most of the vitamins. The fructose sugars are also more balanced and less concentrated in a whole fruit juice.

Sometimes it may be more practical to use the juice, such as in carrot juice, because the pulp can be very filling. If you are eating carrots or even chopped up carrots be careful of aspiration. Carrots are notorious for "going down the wrong throat" and you may choke on them. Carrot juice may be a much safer alternative in limited quantities.

A popular healthy drink is also a **green drink** made from a variety of green vegetables, including cabbage, sweetened with carrots or beets. For those of you without teeth or with poor quality dentures, whole food juicing is definitely the way to go to get all your nutrients from fruits and vegetables. Get a juicing cookbook that will describe tasty combinations.

Remember, five servings of fruits and vegetables a day, which are recommended, will give you large quantities of B6 and folic acid, shown to reduce heart disease through various studies. Since heart disease is a major component of early death, by increasing your quantities of fruits and vegetables, you are, in effect, reducing your chance of dying early from heart disease from which nearly 20.5 million people in the world die off each year. You may also reduce your chance of dying early from cancer because of the photo-chemicals that are protective for your immune system. At the same time, you are strengthening the building blocks of your bones, connective tissues, organs, brain, and skin.

Yes, those five servings of fruits and vegetables will do you well by increasing your antioxidants, helping to prolong your life and keep you healthy and vigorous.

This Chapter on fruits vegetables and dietary choices was important. It nudged you towards making wiser choices in what you eat. It is good to know why you are doing something instead of just taking some magic pill that you know nothing about. Every human body is slightly different. **This is the only body that we have, so we better make sure we give it the best building blocks possible** in order for it to grow healthy and repair itself when things go wrong. Don't skimp on high quality organically produced food. It's like an investment in the best building materials for your home.

Chapter 9

ON VITAMINS AND HORMONES

Vitamins

This chapter has been simplified in order to be easier understood. For more complex and detailed explanations on how specific vitamins, herbs and anti-oxidants work, I would recommend my previous book "Happy Life Healthy Aging" or a book specific to vitamins and minerals written by an expert.

In Nature, everything affects everything. If you take one component out of the system, the entire downstream process is affected. Nature has created a balance through millions of years of adaptation. If that balance is disrupted our biological ecosystem gets thrown out of orbit and starts to self-destruct.

Sometimes our bodies can compensate and sometimes they can't. The ability to compensate is based on our genetic makeup and our diet. The male deer in Shenandoah National Park get selected by the females for breeding by the size of their antlers. The size of their antlers is determined by their genetic makeup and the diet that they have eaten. A healthy nutritious diet will assure antler bone growth of up to a quarter inch per day. If they have a poor diet, their antlers will not grow as much and the females will not select them. They will not be able to propagate their genes.

The food we eat has the same effect on us. It has to be nutritious, with adequate vitamins and minerals in trace amounts in order for us and our offspring to thrive and stay healthy. Doctors do not know exactly what is needed in trace amounts for optimum health and how everything interacts.

If you were stranded on a tropical island and you had the opportunity to take only one vitamin or nutrient with you, which would you take to give you the greatest protective effect and let you live healthy?

Most people would probably say vitamin C and that would be a good choice. However, on a tropical island, you'd most likely have plenty of fruits. Fruits are generally fairly high in vitamin C, so you could get all the vitamin C you need. I would probably select a good multi vitamin, multi mineral combination.

The Vitamin C explanation, from my previous book "Happy Life Healthy Aging", is included below. If you are interested in detailed explanations of other nutrients, you may enjoy reading chapter 6 "Vitamins, Minerals, Herbs and Anti-Oxidants".

Vitamin C

I guess we will start with the most famous of the vitamins, which probably **gives you the biggest bang for the buck**. Going back in my memory banks, I remember when I was a resident studying this vitamin. I was very much interested in natural approaches toward healing even then. I would see these severely emaciated patients come in. Some were very old and had a large number of **pressure sores and ulcerations** around their bodies. The open sores left the patients exposed to massive infections, which would lead to death fairly rapidly.

These people were sent to the rehabilitative center after being in a regular hospital and then progressively getting worse because they had no nutrient reserves. Whenever they were laid on a bed, their skin broke down and became ulcerated.

The standard treatment at the time was force-feeding them Ensure, a chemical nutrient formula designed to sustain life. We fed some of them through a tube in their throat, and in others, a tube was embedded through their abdominal wall. The results were not as satisfying as I had hoped.

I started looking into vitamin C. In the medical library I found a book written in the thirties about vitamin C and all the research done from the turn of the century to the 1930's. I was amazed at the wealth of information that existed on this vitamin so many years ago and shocked that the medical community rarely utilized the information in their treatment protocols.

Medicine knew that ascorbic acid would prevent scurvy, a disease that caused the deaths of many sailors on long voyages, because their diet was short on essential nutrients. However, **medicine rarely used the basic science information that was available as early as 1920 in treatment protocols.** (Nobel laureate Otto Warburg, a Jewish Nazi era scientist in Germany, did groundbreaking cancer metabolism research in 1930s that is only now being re discovered.)

Perhaps one of the reasons that early research was ignored was that drug companies became powerful and infectious diseases had a priority in research; and, the business aspect of medicine was driven by drugs and high-tech surgery.

After presenting the data to my supervisors, I started an **intravenous drip with vitamin C in high concentrations**. I did that on a daily basis. To the surprise of the nursing staff, the severely debilitated patients began to improve fairly rapidly. Their **open lesions healed and their pressure sores reduced in size.**

I had read some of the research done by **Linus Pauling** and his theory of vitamin C. I knew he was taking about 12 to 14 grams of vitamin C per day. I take higher doses of Vitamin C in a powdered form mixed in orange or cranberry juice along with multivitamins and vitamin E, if I feel I'm getting a little under the weather.

I gave the patients **vitamin C** because I knew it was **essential for collagen formation, which is the connective component of the skin and gives the skin elasticity**. When we don't have that elasticity, the skin becomes very thin and breaks down. This elasticity is necessary for all our organs.

There is a condition called scleroderma where patients' skin and connective tissue become very hard and eventually they can't move their hands. Their facial skin becomes real firm, and eventually their digestive track and swallowing mechanism become impaired so they can't swallow.

At the time I was giving intravenous **vitamin C** to my patients, I didn't know of its **importance as an antioxidant and a fighter of free radicals.** When that data emerged, intravenous vitamin C become an important component in the chelation therapy regiment.

Linus Pauling was a good example of the effect of high dose vitamin C. From my understanding, he was mentally clear and in good health until his death in his nineties. He also rarely suffered from infectious diseases because he had a fairly strong immune system. His book, **Vitamin C and the Common Cold**, became a classic and popularized the use of vitamin C for preventative reasons

When **Dr. Harmon** came up with the **theory of free radicals** and described it in detail, vitamin C started taking on a very important role as an antioxidant and nutrient.

As we get older, we slowly shrivel up and bake ourselves to death, like a plum in an oven that becomes a prune or a chicken that turns brown as it bakes. Our skin slowly gets browner, gets more spots, discolors, gets cancer cells, and shrivels up.

This slow damage is caused by free radicals and the oxidation reactions that slowly destroy us.

Oxidation occurs throughout our entire environment. It is evident as rust on metal or a white powder on aluminum. Metal, if it oxidizes enough, eventually breaks down completely. Just leave a piece of metal exposed to the elements and the rust becomes so severe that everything falls apart.

However, if you add phosphoric acid on the metal, the rust is changed biochemically into a coating that protects the metal.

When I was at L'Anse Aux Meadows Newfoundland where the Vikings had a colony 500 years before Columbus discovered America, I noticed the blacksmith shop made a lot of iron nails for their ship's hull. The nails that held the wood planks together constantly had to be coated with tar and eventually replaced because they rusted or oxidized. The Viking boats would fall apart with rusty nails, so they did preventive maintenance.

If the Vikings did preventive maintenance 1000 years ago, shouldn't we at least be thinking about it also?

In the human biological system, you add antioxidants, which inhibit the oxidative reactions occurring to our body. The more antioxidants you take and the more variety of antioxidants you take, theoretically, the slower should will be your aging because you will not shrivel up internally or externally as rapidly.

Vitamin C in high concentrations is also a chelating agent and helps bind toxic metals in our systems, just like EDTA does. In higher concentrations, it has a double effect of decreasing oxidation, keeping us from rusting and shriveling, and eliminating waste. A friend of mine used high dose Vitamin C in powdered form as a laxative, because in high dosages it will cause loose stools.

So what are some of the other benefits attributed to vitamin C based on research data? Vitamin C helps produce collagen, which makes connective tissue stronger. It is known as the cellular glue, and it keeps our tissues from falling apart. A good example is the British sailors aboard ships who developed scurvy. Their symptoms were spongy gums, loose teeth, and bleeding into the skin and mucous membranes. Their cellular connective substance, the glue that holds all our tissues together, fell apart.

The sailors literally fell apart and bled to death because they lacked the cellular connective substance, which is essential and dependent on vitamin C. They also fell over dead, dying of sudden cardiac death because Vitamin C is also essential for heart function.

With **increased vitamin C**, this cellular connective substance builds a **stronger connective tissue**, making the body more resistant to a large host of organisms. A number of studies have demonstrated the benefits of high doses of vitamin C and cancer of the mouth, throat, larynx, stomach, bladder, pancreas, breasts, skin, cervix, colon, rectum, and so on. This anti-cancer effect was well documented by **Dr. Linus Pauling's book, Cancer and Vitamin C.**

In 2015 The National Cancer Institute stated on their web site that: quote.

- Vitamin C is a nutrient found in food and dietary supplements. It is an antioxidant and also plays a key role in making collagen .
- High-dose vitamin C may be given by intravenous (IV) infusion (through a vein into the bloodstream) or orally (taken by mouth). When taken by intravenous infusion, vitamin C can reach much higher levels in the blood than when the same amount is taken by mouth.
- High-dose vitamin C has been studied as a treatment for patients with cancer since the 1970s.
- Laboratory studies have shown that high doses of vitamin C may slow the growth and spread of prostate, pancreatic, liver, colon, and other types of cancer cells.
- Some laboratory and animal studies have shown that combining vitamin C with anticancer therapies may be helpful, while other studies have shown that certain forms of vitamin C may make chemotherapy less effective.
- Animal studies have shown that high-dose vitamin C treatment blocks tumor growth in certain models of pancreatic, liver, prostate, and ovarian cancers, sarcoma, and malignant mesothelioma.
- Some human studies of high-dose IV vitamin C in patients with cancer have shown improved quality of life, as well as improvements in physical, mental, and emotional functions, symptoms of fatigue, nausea and vomiting, pain, and appetite loss.
- Intravenous high-dose ascorbic acid has caused very few side effects in clinical trials.
- While generally approved as a dietary supplement, the U.S. Food and Drug Administration (FDA) has not approved the use of IV high-dose vitamin C as a treatment for cancer or any other medical condition.

The mechanisms and details are beyond the scope of this book, other than to make you aware that vitamin C is an extremely potent protector of our connective tissues. It neutralizes a number of carcinogens, including pesticides, nitrites, nitrosamines, hydrocarbons, air pollutants, industrial chemicals, and so forth. Remember, I told you earlier that vitamin C in high doses is also a potent chelating agent. It helps remove toxic elements from your body.

Another benefit of vitamin C is that it enhances T-lymphocytes, which are the blood components in the immune system that help kill cancer cells. The stronger your immune system, the greater your ability to fight a large host of organisms. Vitamin C has also been found to be beneficial to people with cataracts and helped prevent cataracts in rats. Asthma symptoms have also been reduced by the intake of vitamin C supplementation.

The intensity of a common cold has been decreased by high doses of vitamin C and, also, people don't get colds as frequently when they take high doses of vitamin C, as was exhibited by Dr. Linus Pauling.

Sperm quality, especially in heavy smokers, has been improved by higher dosages of vitamin C. In a 2006 research article sperm count was increased and sperm mobility was significantly increased by taking 1000 mg vitamin C twice daily for 2 months. Vitamin C has shown anti-candida effect. Serum cholesterol has dropped with administrations of one gram of vitamin C. Platelet adhesiveness and platelet aggregation, have been decreased with vitamin C therefore reducing blood clotting.

Other studies showed that six weeks of vitamin C supplementation lowered pulse and systolic blood pressure in patients with borderline hypertension. A Japanese study in terminal cancer patients showed an increased survival time of up to five times longer with patients given vitamin C versus the non-vitamin C patients.

The evidence goes on and on with a host of worldwide studies showing the benefits of vitamin C.

As you can see, vitamin C is an effective immune enhancing agent, increasing your resistance. It is a potent scavenger of free radicals, which cause you to age and shrivel away.

The studies on vitamin C are too numerous to elaborate on, but the data have been available since the thirties when the original studies were made on guinea pigs with the promotion of wound healing by the use of vitamin C and its requirement for collagen synthesis. The free radical and anti-aging benefits of vitamin C have only recently been recognized since free radicals have been implicated in our aging process and disease process.

For how many years have you heard sunscreen, sunscreen, sunscreen for the prevention of skin cancers, some of these skin cancers can be deadly. In a recent meeting of the American College of Dermatology, new findings came to light. Although the American population had been using high amounts of sunscreen, the skin cancer rate remained the same or increased. If sunscreens were to protect against skin cancer, they certainly didn't do a good job. It appears that all they managed to do was protect against sunburn.

The newest theory is that the free radical damage to our skin actually caused the cancer. Now, they recommend high dosages of antioxidants, to include multiple servings of fruits and vegetables daily. I find that to be an interesting shift in focus from chemical drugs and surgical treatment to a preventative approach.

So, what does all this have to do with longevity?

If you have a healthy immune system and fewer diseases, you'll have a greater chance of living longer.

The less sick you are, the greater will be your ability to enjoy life to its fullest, even at an old age.

Reducing free radical damage to your system, be it the skin, brain, arterial system, plaque buildup, or cancers, will greatly enhance your chances to survive into old age. It certainly makes sense to me that vitamin C is a good preventative measure to take in your anti-aging program.

Nutrition minded doctors recommend 1000 to 3000 mg of the ester vitamin C. I personally like taking the powdered form of vitamin C because it is easy to take; it mixes with juice, and gives me a high dose fairly rapidly. The bioflavonoids, which are extremely important, are obtained through my multivitamin, as well as the fruits and vegetables I eat.

Dosage ranges of various supplements used in Anti-Aging

(Mostly derived from Michael Janson M.D. Longevity Medicine Supplement lectures at the ACAM anti-aging courses.)

It is advisable that the higher dosages be taken only under **supervision of a physician familiar with the nutrient.**

Vitamin A 10,000 IU to 50,000 IU. You need to be cautious with pregnancy if you take more than 10,000

IU or 3,000 micrograms/d since birth defects may occur as well as liver damage in some people. (One microgram equals 3.33 international units (IU))

Carotenoids 15,000 to 50,000 IU, preferably mixed carotenoids rather than beta-carotene alone.

Vitamin B1 50 mg to 500 mg. (Thiamine)

Vitamin B2 50 mg to 500 mg. (Riboflavin)

Vitamin B3 50 mg to 3000 mg, taken as (Niacin, Niacinamide, or Inositol Hexaniacinate.)

Vitamin B5 100 mg to 2000 mg, as (Pantothenic acid or calcium pantothenate). By the way, 900 mg pantethene in a coenzyme form of pantothenate appears to lower cholesterol

Vitamin B6 50 mg to 300 mg daily. (Pyridoxine) However, in high dosages of 500 mg to 6,000 mg you may get neuropathy, so the dosage needs to be monitored.

Vitamin B12 100 mcg to 1000 mcg daily. (Cyanocobalamine) People often take the higher dosage in intramuscular injections as hydroxycobalamin.

Folic acid 800 mcg to 80,000 mcg. At 80 mg, it has been used for gout. In pregnancy, 1 mg to 5 mg is used. 5 mg is a common folic acid dosage.

Vitamin C 2 grams to 50 grams, either oral, intravenous, or combinations. That may sound like a high dosage. Some people take about 4-5 grams a day in a powdered from in juice. People have used these high dosages successfully as an IV drip, especially in fighting fatal diseases. 1-2 grams in pill form is more common for general use.
Vitamin D 200 to 400 IU, older people may need the higher dose. A short 15 min walk in the sun will be just as effective.

Vitamin E 400 IU to 3,000 IU, preferably in a mixed state, as previously mentioned, of alpha, beta, delta, and gamma. It has to be a natural form of vitamin E. Synthetic vitamin E, d-l-Alpha tocopherol generally should not exceed 800 IU. The natural form has been taken at the higher dosages.

Coenzyme Q10 100 mg to 400 mg; occasionally higher, up to 600 mg. It is taken in oil-based or lecithin chewable forms.

Magnesium 500 mg to 1,000 mg. Magnesium has a calming effect on muscles, agitation and anxiety. It helps with constipation and is often used as a natural sleep aid.

Calcium 500 mg to 1,000 mg.

Chromium 200 mcg to 1,200 mcg. The higher dosages are used in diabetes.

Selenium 200 mcg to 1,000 mcg. Again, the higher dosages are sometimes used in disease states.

Zinc 15 mg to 80 mg. It is used in combination of 10:1 or 15:1 with copper.

Copper 2 mg to 5 mg.

Manganese 10 mg to 20 mg.

L-glutamine 2 grams to 8 grams. (It can be absorbed through the blood brain barrier) It is also given in combination with ginkgo biloba for memory.

L-carnitine 500 mg to 2,000 mg.

Taurine 1,000 mg to 3,000 mg. Taurine has been found to be beneficial in maintaining retinal function and it is sometimes added to the intravenous chelation drip for people with macular degeneration. Taurine has also been used experimentally on rabbits with induced congestive heart failure and found to be beneficial.

Mixed Bioflavonoids 1,000 mg to 4,000 mg

Quercetin 800 mg to 1,600 mg. Quercetin is used as an anti-inflammatory and anti-allergic agent and appears to inhibit histamine release which decreases inflammation.

Ginkgo Biloba 120 mg to 240 mg at 24% standardized extract.

Proanthocyanidins OPC 50 mg to 200 mg, usually as a grape seed extract or pine bark extract, sometimes a mixture of both plus red wine extract, citrus peel extract and bilberry extract. Many people feel Pycnogenol may be an even more potent antioxidant than vitamins E and C.

Silymarin (milk thistle) extract 150 mg to 600 mg of 80% standardized extract. This is obtained from the seed shell of the milk thistle, which contains powerful bioflavonoid-like chemicals, used to protect the liver and rebuild damaged cells, such as in hepatitis, cirrhosis, and jaundice. Alpha Lipoic Acid, Selenium and Silymarin have been used successfully for Hepatitis C.

Echinacea 250 mg to 1,000 mg of mixed standardized extract. Echinacea has been used as a powerful natural antibiotic by many people.

Garlic 500 mg to 2,000 mg of deodorized powder. I personally prefer natural garlic, crushed on garlic toast, which I use at the earliest onset of cold symptoms.
Saw palmetto 320 mg to 640 mg of standardized extract. Saw palmetto has been used effectively for prostatic hypertrophy. People that use it, love it.

Bilberry 100 mg to 300 mg of 15% to 25% standardized anthocyanosides content. Bilberry has been shown to have vaso-protective and anti-edema effects in animal trials (protects blood vessels and swelling). It has also been shown to reduce ischemia (lack of blood supply) damage.

Melatonin 0.5 mg to 6 mg at bedtime. Melatonin is a very important hormone that has been used for insomnia and jet lag. The most important part of melatonin is that it is a potent antioxidant and protects against free radical damage.

This is an incomplete list of vitamins, minerals, and supplements.

Below are the dosages of the multivitamin – mineral supplements we used in our Chelation Medical Centers practice. Dosages are per serving.

"**cMc**" Multi-Vitamin, Mineral, Trace Element Supplements

Vitamin A (Palmitate)	10,000 I.U.
Vitamin A (Beta Carotene Vitamin A Activity)	10,000 I.U.
Vitamin C (L-Ascorbic Acid Corn Free)	1,200 mg
Vitamin D-3 (Cholecalciferol)	200 I.U.
Vitamin E (d-Alpha Tocopheryl Succinate)	400 I.U.
Vitamin B-1 (Thiamine Mononitrate)	100 mg
Vitamin B-2 (Riboflavin)	50 mg
Vitamin B-3 (Niacin)	50 mg
Vitamin B-3 (Niacinamide)	150 mg
Vitamin B-6 (Pyridoxine HCL)	25 mg

Folic Acid (Folacin)	800 mcg
Vitamin B-12 (On ion Exchange Resin)	150 mcg
Biotin	300 mcg
Pantothenic Acid (d-Calcium Pantothenate)	350 mg
Calcium (Citrate)	500 mg
Iodine (Kelp)	200 mcg
Magnesium (Ascorbate, Aspartate, Gluconate and Oxide)	500 mg
Zinc (Gluconate Aspartate)	25 mg
Selenium (Amino Acid Complex Selenemax)	200 mcg
Manganese (Gluconate Aspartate)	25 mg
Copper (Amino Acid Chelate)	2 mg
Chromium (Amino Acid Chelate)	200 mcg
Molybdenum (Amino Acid Chelate)	100 mcg
Potassium (Gluconate Aspartate)	99 mg
Boron (Aspartate-Citrate)	1000 mcg
Choline (Bitartrate)	100 mg
Citrus Bioflavonoids	150 mg
Inositol	100 mg
PABA (Para Amino Benzoic Acid)	100 mg
Vanadium (Amino Acid Chelate)	30 mcg

Stearic Acid, Microcrystalline Cellulose, Croscarmellose Sodium, Hydroxypropyl Cellulose, Magnesium Stearate, Silicon Dioxide, Ethylcellulose and Sodium Lauryl Sulfate

You can get really carried away with supplementation and be taking hundreds of pills a day. For most people, this basic list of C, E, B-complex, selenium, along with good multivitamins and trace minerals, should be adequate for antioxidant protection. Some people often want to add OPCs to the supplement list due to their potent antioxidant effects. The **list of supplement** dosages is meant **only as a reference point** for you when you check the content of your multivitamin and mineral supplements. This list gives you some sort of basis to go by in evaluating the potency of the supplements you are taking.

As you can see from this extensive list supplements can become quite confusing, as to dosages and types taken. A healthy diet of colored fruits and vegetables, at five servings a day, will give you many of the essential minerals and vitamins you need. However, due to the free radical damage that is occurring through all the pollutants in our environment, extra supplements may be needed as insurance, and the potent antioxidants, vitamins and minerals as described in this chapter are a good way to start in protecting yourself from oxidative stress and micronutrient depletion.

Take a clue from nature... Oxford University researchers observed Chimpanzees in the Uganda Budongo Forest eating kaolinite clay to detoxify and boost their mineral content. The long term study published on PLOS ONE in 2015 described how the mineral source for the chimps (raffia palm leaves) has diminished so they started supplementing their diet with clay. Do the chimps know something that we don't?

On a tropical island, I would take a multi vitamin, multi mineral vitamin pill similar to the one we used in our clinics. Above was the breakdown of its content.

ON HORMONES

Chapter 7 in my previous book "Happy Life Healthy" has an extensive section on hormones in it. How selective hormones work in your body and why they are necessary. Hormones are pharmacological and need to be handled by a physician. This book is designed to show you what you can do for yourself. If you wish to find out more on how they work, you may want to read my previous book or a book specifically designed for that purpose.

The more naturally you can increase hormones, the better, such as through vigorous physical exercise, as I discussed previously. However, sometimes supplementation is needed. If you decide to use high dosages of hormone precursors, I recommend having your hormone levels monitored either by blood tests or saliva tests, and also have your intake monitored by a qualified physician. Flax seeds sprinkled on fruit or cereal, are an easy way to supplement all the essential fatty acids our body needs for hormonal production.

Now for the bad news: Researchers very recently discovered a "switch" in the round worm, a commonly studied species. Once the reproductive phase is over, this switch turns on which starts the aging process. In humans it's the decrease of Growth Hormone, Estrogen, Testosterone and other hormones. The Telomeres on our chromosomes get shorter, we get shorter, and our mind gets filled up with tangles and so on. Every cell in our body has programmed cell death, called apoptosis. For every action there is an equal and opposite reaction, a law of Physics. Be careful what you put into your body and mind.

My goal in this book is to get you stimulated to start your healthy aging and longevity journey. You never get anywhere unless you take the first step and start. I want every fellow baby boomer to have the best retirement possible and to enjoy the fruits of their labor without physical impediments. You just want to place the odds in your favor, and that is what this book is about.

Chapter 10

Self Help Aging Test

It's nice to have some kind of objective criteria as to how well we are aging physiologically. We know our chronological age, how old we are, but do we know our physiological age? Your physiological age is determined by how well your body functions. There are the young old and the old old. Both groups of people may have the same chronological age but different physiological age. On my world cruise, some 75 year olds are using the walker while others are walking up 9 floors of stairs just to go to the cafeteria for breakfast. There is obviously going to be a difference in both sets of individuals in their physiological age even though they are at the same numerical age. Your physiological age can be kept track of accurately by a few objective tests that you can do at home. Have someone assist you so you don't fall.

Equipment needed

1. A grip strength device ... also called a hand dynamometer. Personally I prefer the old fashioned flat metal elliptical kind that is fat in the middle and tapers on both ends. It has a pointer in the middle of the elliptical ring like a clock hand. The pointer goes to the right on a scale that tells you how many pounds of pressure you have exerted by squeezing the device. It is mechanical and less prone to failure. I used it in my practice for years. We also had hydraulic hand dynamometers where you squeezed two handles together, but, those were more prone to failure.

2. A simple wooden or metal 1 foot ruler. You can also use a wooden yard stick or a metric 1 meter stick.

3. A stop watch or timing device that you can use with one hand.

That's all you need in order to objectively measure your chronological age progress for the better or for the worse. If you decide to do many of the suggestions in this book, your objective criteria of your physiological age should improve. Keep all of the above equipment in "my aging box" along with a small notebook which will have your name and the date the tests were done.

#1 Grip Strength is a good indicator of your overall health, it decreases with age. It is the power that you can exert by squeezing something hard. Take your hand dynamometer and squeeze it 3 times with each hand. Record the date, time of day and the foot pounds of pressure that the dial measured. The pointer should stay on the maximum pounds after you squeezed. Every time you squeeze the dynamometer record your finding. You will have six readings in your notebook labeled ... Right hand #1, #2, #3 and Left hand #1, #2, #3 under a particular date. This becomes your objective data that you can track over time. You can do this test every six months if you wish. It is objective and does not lie just like your scale doesn't lie about your weight.

#2 The Ruler Pinch test.... This test measures your hand reflexes. It is a simple test that is objective. Your reflexes are important in preventing injuries. If you can reflexively respond to a slip or tripping over something then you may be able to prevent injury. This test also measures how fast your nervous system responds.

Take the ruler and hold it between your thumb and your index finger upright at the base. You will be holding the ruler upright at the 1 inch or one centimeter mark.

Briefly open your thumb and index finger and let the ruler drop between your fingers but immediately close your finger and thumb together again in a pinching motion to stop the ruler from falling. You will see on the ruler where your fingers are and record that figure. If you start out at 1 inch, open and close your fingers rapidly, and the ruler is now at six inches when you pinched your fingers together, you will record 6 inches or 10 centimeters.

Do this ruler pinch test 3 times with each hand and record your findings just like you did with the grip strength test.

#3 The Balance Test ... have a stopwatch in one had that you can start with the push of a button. Stand behind a couch, a large living room chair or next to a bed. You need to be next to something that you can grab to prevent falling.

Standing with your feet together, simultaneously start the stop watch and raise your left leg forward and see how long you can balance yourself on one leg. The second that you touch ground with the raised leg, stop the stop watch and record the number of seconds on the watch. If you are about to fall, put your foot down and grab the couch to prevent falling.

Do this test three times on one leg, each time recording your time on the stop watch. After you finish one leg, face the opposite direction and do this same balance stability test with the other leg. You will have 3 measurement of time for the right leg and 3 measurements for the left leg.

The "Tandem walk test" is another balance test that you could do is to see how far you can walk on a straight line placing one foot exactly in front of the other with your heel of one foot touching the toes of the other. Get a tape measure and measure that distance after each attempt.

This test will become harder and harder to do as you age. Record your distance walked on that straight line doing it three times.

The final test that you may also want to do is a simple memory test. Before you do the above physiologic tests, grab a book, open it up to a page and randomly place your finger on a page. Record which word is over your finger and write it down in your notebook on back side of your data recording page. Repeat that process on another page and write down the word over your finger. Do this a third, fourth or fifth time and write down the words. Try to remember the words.

Do the physiologic tests mentioned above and then under all of your test results write down the 3 5 or 10 words that you remembered. Flip your page over to see how accurate you were and give yourself a score such as 3/5. That means that you remembered three words out of five which is a 60% score.

These simple objective home tests of your physiological age are a good general indicator of your bodies aging. How are your numbers doing year after year? Are they staying the same, improving or getting worse? How about your random memory test? How many words can you remember?

Hopefully if you chose to work on staying healthy and becoming the young old, all the above test number should not decline very much and some may even improve.

Good Luck

CHAPTER 11

EXPERIMENTAL AGENTS FOR LIFE EXTENSION

For a long time I debated if to include anything about chemical agents in this book. There are a number of gerontology researchers and individuals taking all kinds of compounds and drugs trying to prolong their lives. Once one pathway is discovered, people jump on it thinking that that is the magic bullet. A compound that will allow them to live longer. If side effects are discovered they will jump on something else. Chemical alterations of natural biological processes is very tricky and can be dangerous to your health. Below is a list of agents some experimenters are taking for longevity. I personally do not endorse them and believe that nature has developed a fine balance for the preservation of the human species.

So what agents are gerontology research groups trying out in order to try to prolong their lives?

Metformin – is a drug used for management of type 2 diabetes. It has been available for a long time and is the most prescribed agent to try to control diabetes. The theory in its use in longevity is that if you keep blood sugars low, you will have less stress on your system and less inflammation. There is a clinical trial going on called TAME, Targeting Aging with Metformin that is investigating this medication. Over many years of use, it has been noticed that people taking metformin had a lower cancer rate, lower death rate and better health. How do we know that it is metformin, or just not having elevated blood sugar in your system? Diabetes is related to cancer as well as a host of diseases.

Rapamycin – is an immunosuppressive drug used in organ transplantation. The molecule was originally found on Easter Island, where the Moai statues are, in a bacteria known as Streptomyces Hygroscopicus. The drug Rapamycin was developed from that bacteria. It prevents your body from attacking a transplanted organ. It apparently has had some benefit in mammalian life span extension. Male and female mice lived longer on Rapamycin. The belief is that low doses of rapamycin taken intermittently may prolong life span. There are books devoted to this unique drug.

Resveratrol – a compound discovered in red wine. This compound has multiple benefits as an antioxidant, anti-inflammatory, immunomodulatory agent. It helps regulate glucose and lipid metabolism. It is neuroprotective, cancer protective and Alzheimer's protective. It extended the lifespan of metabolically compromised mice but does not always extend lifespan. You would have to become an alcoholic to get enough of it by drinking wine.

Acarbose – is a type 2 diabetic medication just like metformin is. It has extended the life expectancy of mice through affecting the gut bacteria. It has also been used for weight loss.

17 alpha estradiol – Alfatradiole, the brand name, is male sex specific, it has extended survival rate in experimental male animals by 19% but not in female animals.

Gene editing – something in the future. Editing out genes that eventually cause senescence or failure of cell replication.

Young Plasma – young plasma from young blood appears to rejuvenate blood DNA methylation profile. It extends mean lifespan and appearance of older rats. It apparently contains elements that seem to prolong life in older test animals.

After a time, we may find out that all those chemical interventions are just pipe dreams. Our biological system is far more complicated than we ever envisioned. Nature has evolved over millions of years. You are part of nature, if you cheat nature you cheat yourself.

Conclusion

How we age is a choice, a choice you make every day to stay mentally and physically functional. Healthy aging requires work, but the rewards are well worth it.

Healthy aging is your job in retirement, take it seriously.

May you be successful in your quest for a long, happy and healthy retirement.

Best Wishes

Dr. John P. Lenhart

If you think information in this book was helpful, please write a review. Thanks

References: www.happylifehealthyaging.com

About the author:

John P Lenhart MD DC, is board certified in Physical Medicine and Rehabilitation with years of experience in Orthopedic and Rehabilitative Medicine. He has been a lecturer at international conferences, interviewed on Television and has written several books on anti-aging. Dr. Lenhart is one of the few physicians in the world that has training in Medicine, Acupuncture, Chiropractic, Applied Kinesiology, Chelation and Nutrition. He used an integrative and complementary approach to treating patients throughout his entire medical career. He believes that there is a time and place for every aspect of medicine.

Made in the USA
Monee, IL
04 November 2026

67374647R00148